The International Lib

THE PERSON IN
PSYCHOLOGY

Founded by C. K. Ogden

The International Library of Psychology

GENERAL PSYCHOLOGY
In 38 Volumes

THE PERSON IN PSYCHOLOGY

Reality or Abstraction

PAUL LAFITTE

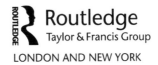

LONDON AND NEW YORK

First published in 1957 by
Routledge and Kegan Paul Ltd
2 Park Square, Milton Park, Abingdon, Oxfordshire OX14 4RN
711 Third Avenue, New York, NY 10017

First issued in paperback 2014

Routledge is an imprint of the Taylor and Francis Group, an informa business

British Library Cataloguing in Publication Data
A CIP catalogue record for this book
is available from the British Library

The Person in Psychology
ISBN 978-0415-21030-0
General Psychology: 38 Volumes
ISBN 0415-21129-8
The International Library of Psychology: 204 Volumes
ISBN 0415-19132-7

ISBN 13: 978-1-138-87531-9 (pbk)
ISBN 13: 978-0-415-21030-0 (hbk)

CONTENTS

CONTENTS

FOREWORD

BY O. A. OESER
PROFESSOR OF PSYCHOLOGY, UNIVERSITY OF MELBOURNE

THIS book states a hypothesis about the nature of psychological enquiry and the proper field of psychology. Consequently it takes issue with the major problems of methodology and theory in the various branches and schools of psychology, with many of which it stands at diameter and sword's point.

When, about the middle of the nineteenth century, the science of experimental psychology was born, the infant was crippled by an array of physical and physiological instruments. It was starved on a diet of psychophysics and later of rats. Put less metaphorically, for close on a century psychologists refused to regard the person as an appropriate unit on which to focus their studies. Only the psycho-analytic schools tried to understand the person, his determinations and his historical engagement with the world. They also made inductive generalizations on the basis of which attempts could be made to change the person. It is only in the past twenty years that this one-sided approach has been broadened and that the study of the social psychology of personality has been taking the lead.

Much thought is at present being devoted to the nature and implications of a unified social or behavioural science, to new conceptual syntheses of psychology, philosophy, anthropology and sociology. Lafitte somewhere uses the term 'philosophical anthropology' and thus re-introduces psychologists to a stream of thinking which started with the Greeks, was given the name by von Humboldt and reappeared in the works of Erich Jaensch before it was dried up by the upsurge of a barbaric and anti-scientific power mythology. At the centre of this unified science of behaviour is the person in his involvement with himself and his societies. He is what Lafitte persuades us to regard as the proper object and focus of psychology.

He makes a sustained attack on many of the present suppositions, methods and pre-occupations of psychology, and follows this with a sustained constructive argument and exposition as to remedies. This may be irritating or even exasperating to some. I am reminded, however, that organisms act on stimuli. Voltaire wrote a serious poem and an extended literary fantasy to scarify the perverters of the philosophy of Leibniz, and Voltaire's stimulus had a most salutary effect. The perversions or pseudo-sciences of some psychometricians, psychoanalysts and rat lovers are seriously, but none the less devastatingly, dealt with by Lafitte. I have no doubt that this will prove to be a most valuable stimulus to clarify thinking about psychological theory.

Whether or not the reader agrees with Lafitte's definition and delimitation of the field of psychology, there is no doubt that this book fills a gap in the literature of psychology. It also satisfies the need for a thorough review of its methods and their implications in the wider setting of all the sciences of man. And it fits perfectly into the present trend towards review and conceptual clarification in theoretical psychology.

Lafitte tries to see psychology as a whole, as a science in its own right quite independent of physics or biochemistry or biology; to review the meaning, purpose and significance of its methodological equipment. I would confidently place this book in the hands of every advanced student of psychology and of all others who are interested in the study of man. Even if the latter lack the extensive conceptual and experimental training required of a modern psychologist, they will benefit from the reading and enjoy it, provided they are prepared for hard thinking and intensive learning.

PREFACE

A BOOK which is, in effect, a general argument about the nature of psychology hardly needs a preface except to explain features in the presentation of the argument that might otherwise appear strange.

One of these features is the fairly frequent reference made to the ideas of various philosophers. In principle, this is not remarkable. Every psychologist makes philosophical presuppositions in the course of his work, whether or not he knows he is doing so, and psychologists sometimes even state and discuss their presuppositions. Nor does it matter that the philosophers referred to are, for the most part, not at all the kind of persons one would usually find in company with empirical psychology. It may matter, however, that the argument is set out by an applied psychologist with no professional competence in philosophy. It would have been preferable to leave the task to a psychologist with philosophical training or to a philosopher with a training in empirical psychology. But that might have meant leaving it indefinitely, and it therefore seemed better to undertake the task now and to insert this warning to the reader.

Somewhat the same applies to my periodical references to cases and especially to the extensive references to the results of work in progress (chiefly, but not solely, my own) in Chapters 7, 9, 10, 11 and 12. I do not for a moment suppose that my professional experience is of any special importance, but it seems inevitable that one should refer to what lies readiest to hand. Where this includes reference to quite complex unpublished findings, it is bound to be unsatisfactory to the reader who cannot refer to the original. However, I feel that it would have been even less satisfactory to leave the argument unsupported by any detailed evidence. The alternative would have been to leave it till work now in hand was completed. But this again might have meant indefinite postponement, for any psychologist who is fortunate enough to be able to combine teaching, practice and research is bound to have more work in hand than he can ever expect to finish. In this connection I acknowledge with gratitude the permission of Professor O. A. Oeser to refer to certain unpublished work of his own, on job preferences (in Chapters 7 and 9), and to the interim results of a departmental industrial investigation (in Chapters 9, 10, 11 and 12).

I am generally indebted to my colleagues in two ways. Many particular points in the argument have been suggested, and many difficulties clarified, by conversations in the ordinary course of daily work; and the help I have thus received is so extensive that I could not acknowledge it in detail without writing a preface of inordinate length. More important than this are the variety of experience and development in comprehension which have been given me by my working for the past nine years in a Department with a wide range of activities in the community, a stimulating diversity of interests and opinions and a sustained high level of intellectual discussion. For this experience I shall always be indebted to all my colleagues in this period, and above all to the head of the Department.

PAUL LAFITTE

Department of Psychology
University of Melbourne

INTRODUCTION

LIKE many abstract words, psychology has several meanings. In popular usage it may mean the person's ordinary conduct of his affairs and it does mean this when he has done something ingenious or subtle and so thinks of himself as a bit of a psychologist. For the philosopher, psychology is the categorical study of human behaviour; the logical analysis of what people universally and necessarily do. The psychologist, if he tries to distinguish the professional sense of the word, might define it as the empirical or scientific study of human behaviour. But this is hardly sufficient to give the word a proprietary sense: the common sense psychologist, on the one hand, is empirical in his degree and the philosopher, on the other hand, must share with the professional psychologist the study of what everybody necessarily does.

The distinction is easily made by describing what the psychologist does. He tests the person's skin resistance, determines his standing on a social distance scale, traces the manifestations of his anal-sadistic tendencies and measures his spatial ability. These procedures are irrelevant to philosophical psychology and are beyond the grasp of common sense psychology. The psychologist uses them, of course, not merely in order to establish his independence but so that he will be able to construct a specialized picture of the object of his study, the person.

In this task also he is successful. For the field theorist, the person is an object in a field of force with a number of magnetic focuses that are screened from each other. For the psychoanalyst, he is a not very intelligently egotistic child who in adult circumstances blindly repeats and continually fails to solve the conflicts of his nursery days. The social psychologist sees the person as a type exemplifying a class or a set of classes. The physiological psychologist sees him as a resonating storage circuit. Lastly, for the general empiricist, or the psychologist who is not attached to a clearly

1

defined school, the person is an intersection in a statistical hyper-space, the dimensions of which are traits, factors, tests, aptitudes or the like.

The psychologist seldom stops to consider that these descriptions bear little resemblance to each other and even less resemblance to the person as he is known by ordinary persons, among these being the psychologist himself when he is off duty. If he does consider these points he might be inclined to answer that they are the inevit-able defects, if indeed they are defects, of a science that is only a few decades old. One might infer that after more investigation, and especially more scientifically designed investigation with exact statis-tical controls, both peculiarities will disappear. If this inference is correct, psychology has only to go on in its present course and nobody need be dissatisfied now, except perhaps the applied psycho-logist who has to fit the peculiarities of his professional knowledge into his practice.

A brief consideration of this practice, however, will show that its considerable difficulties are not all of a kind that could easily be removed by the extension of psychological knowledge. It will be sufficient to take an ordinary case from the field of vocational counselling. A man wants to change his job. He is 23 years old and has been doing much the same kind of routine work in a large office since he left school at the age of 16 after failing the Leaving Certifi-cate. He is quite satisfied with the actual work he does and is indeed proud of the fact that his records are beautifully kept, always accur-ate and always up to date. But the job is a dead end, and he wants a job from which he can rise on his merits to a high executive position. Although he likes routine to the extent of being quite put out if he is asked to do some work out of order, or if some documents are not at hand when due, he is sure he would rise if he had the quali-fications. To get these, he is prepared to undertake part-time study, perhaps in accountancy. He is not very bright. He would not think of marrying until he can have a nice home in a good suburb and can support his wife in the style proper to a lady.

The counsellor will, of course, have much more information than is given in this bald outline but he will still have difficulty enough in the first stage, making a diagnosis. His client wants two things in life, social status and an object-handling job which he can do to perfection; but his intelligence might be inadequate for the further training required for social mobility. The counsellor might take this last point first as it is perhaps the easiest. Referring to the figures showing intelligence against performance in specified accountancy courses, he can make an actuarial prediction of his client's perform-ance. He could make a prediction that includes other variables by asking his client to work through a social aspirations inventory and a job adjustment inventory, or perhaps by giving him a general projective test. The counsellor would probably not be able simply to use a multiple regression that gives him an improved prediction and it may be doubted whether he will ever be able to do this. A prediction of this kind must depend on the use of *ad hoc* instruments that correspond as closely as possible to the particular client's individual drives or goals and that have been tested before against the criterion which the client is proposing to attempt. The proliferation of specific tests in applied psychology, and their use with more and more specific criteria, may both seem endless but both are limited by the time that can be put into their construction and application. However, this is a difficulty of practice, not of principle.

What the counsellor does, then, is to assess his client's prospects by drawing on his experience of similar cases and on his client's report of similar past situations in his education. The counsellor may thus be able to decide whether or not the person's drive for status is strong enough to outweigh the limitations of his intelligence and whether his perfectionism in work will be a handicap or an asset in his proposed course of study. Although this kind of practical judgement is not necessarily unscientific, the counsellor may be a little ashamed of his leaning so heavily on the psychology of common experience. Consoling himself with the thought that, after all, he is only an applied psychologist, he then finds that his troubles are by no means over when he has made this, the easiest, part of the diagnosis.

He has to consider next a possibility that has already been implied: that his client's two main drives, for status and for perfectionism in work, may conflict. The one may spur him on while the other holds him back, whether during his studies or in his work. Even if he gets a formal qualification, the promotion he wants may well depend on his showing himself capable of varying his speed, order of work and standards: which are precisely the things he hates to vary. The difficulty is now not only practical, that there is insufficient information about similar cases. Unless the counsellor is prepared to reduce his client's description of his own drives to a set of test measurements (and so to abandon the greater part of his information) he has to interpret these drives in order to decide what cases are similar: and his interpretation will depend on the school of psychology that he favours.

Thus he may think that his client's style of work is merely a habit, of long standing and therefore strong, but capable of extinction by the systematic practice of a contrary habit, such as working to a deliberately varied routine. Or the person's style may be an autonomous drive with considerable ego-involvement, in which case he

3

will not change it unless he can see that other ways of working would also enhance his ego. Or again, his style may be the disguised expression of recurrent unsolved conflicts over toilet training: and in this case it will be open to appreciable change only by psychoanalysis. The difficulty with the person's drive for social status is similar. This may be a recently learnt evaluation of the structure of his society, by no means of central importance to him and therefore easily capable of change. Or, so far as it expresses a particular kind of object-love (desire for expensive possessions) rather than a desire for social recognition, it may be another expression of his conflicts over toilet training.

This simplified presentation does little justice to the possibilities of the case. Even so, it is clear that there is a wide range. If the counsellor takes the simplest view of his client's drives, he finds no problem, for his client will presumably be reasonably content if he stays where he is without trying for promotion, or even if he tries and fails. On the most complex view the problem is hardly soluble. If the man stays in his present job he will satisfy his desire for order and acquisition only at work: if he achieves a more responsible job he will satisfy this desire in his home at the cost of doing violence to it in his work.

The best the counsellor can do is again to draw on his experience to decide among the possibilities. Having finished his diagnosis, he then has to decide how to handle the case. He has to consider what facts to present to his client and how to discuss them; how far his client will be able to take the lead in sorting out his position and prospects and how far he may have to lead him. Finally, during the counselling session or sessions the counsellor has to change his procedure to suit his client's growing perception of the situation. All these decisions, whether deliberate or immediate, are made on the same basis of experience. This will be backed up by the guided experience of the counsellor's training and may be supplemented by the experience of others, as reported in case studies. It will be little illuminated, however, by psychological theory, for the personal relation in counselling has for the most part been left to common sense psychology to study.

One may well suppose that the counsellor would actually find little difficulty in this case, for his client has nothing to lose by trying his proposed course of action so long as he does so with the clearest picture he can attain of what it will involve. The case is presented so as to illustrate the typical weaknesses of psychology; insufficient facts, sharply conflicting interpretations, neglect of the study of the greater part of common experience and a wide gap between the person of professional psychology and the person as commonly known. It may be that these weaknesses, which are found to some extent in even the simplest selection procedures, let alone in the complex fields of educational and clinical psychology, do not seriously hinder practice in any field. It may be, too, that they will disappear in time. But the progress of psychology depends on where it goes as well as how far it goes: and it is the direction of progress that may need consideration.

THE FUNDAMENTAL ASSUMPTIONS OF PSYCHOLOGY

Concretely, it is possible that the weaknesses of psychology are due not only to its youth but also to the basic assumptions psychologists make about the nature and status of evidence and of lawfulness or explanation in human behaviour. Whether or not these assumptions are made explicitly, they are bound to be closely related to other assumptions about the general characteristics of human behaviour, as known in common experience: and both sets of assumptions might be expected to determine the methods used for handling or studying human behaviour. Now everyone has more or less elaborated methods for these purposes, so that where psychologists differ among themselves in their methods and especially where they differ from common everyday practice, one would expect to find equally marked differences in the general assumptions of either kind.

Differences in methods may be considered first, starting with the simple consideration of what range of information is used in judging and dealing with other persons and oneself. For these purposes, the non-specialist (and the psychologist, off duty) rely almost entirely on ordinary daily behaviour in ordinary real life situations. Psychology is very different. The field theorist, the psychoanalyst and the social psychologist make some use of this kind of evidence, but it is drawn from specially selected, and in some cases specially constructed, situations only. The general empiricist, whether he measures traits or aptitudes or factors, and the physiological psychologist both rely exclusively on behaviour in specially constructed situations, which are mostly remote from real life. There are consequent and equally marked differences in the use made of historical information. Only the psychoanalysts treat this as fully relevant, but even they conceive the person's history much more narrowly than does the person himself. The field theorist and the social psychologist may make a limited comparative use of historical information but for the other kinds of psychology one can only say that although the person does continue, he has no history.

In the handling of raw information there are marked differences among psychologists. The empiricist approach, physiological psychology and to a large extent social psychology all use measurements of behaviour which is uniformly extended in space or time or which, more usually, can be made so by the use of the elaborate conventional devices of 'measurement theory'. Field theory, in its phenomenal interpretation of the person's situation, is close to common experience in making no attempt to treat behaviour as dimensional in the physical sense, though the symbolic system of the pure field theorists is remote from common expression. Psychoanalysis is similarly close to common experience in its naïve acceptance of behaviour as it is reported, although its translation of this behaviour into the terms of a special system is far removed from the more superficial common experience.

With regard to the general handling of the experimental situation, the differences within psychology are naturally slight, as the purpose of any psychology is to study the person objectively. In common experience, personal relations in which both parties or all parties are more or less deeply involved emotionally are frequent and the relation of pure information-giving or seeking is a special case found only in casual and fleeting contacts. The techniques of psychology are all designed to reduce every relation to this special case, though they differ among themselves. The psychoanalyst's training is the most elaborate technique and some other therapists, together with some social psychologists (such as 'participant observers') have also given detailed consideration to the problem of maintaining their neutrality. For the empiricist and the physiological psychologist there is no problem so long as instructions or questions are unambiguously worded.

There is a similar division in psychology's treatment of the individual case. For social psychology, physiological psychology and general empiricism the individual is an instance of general laws, which can fail to account for his individuality only in so far as they may have been inadequately formulated. The psychoanalyst and the field theorist do not entirely exclude the possibility that general laws may have to be supplemented by some purely individual laws. In this they make a judgement similar to that of common experience, which depends on types, classes and other generalizations but which is always open to exceptions.

The last method of handling human behaviour that requires notice is the most general: the construction of the theories or summary descriptions of the person which were set out at the beginning of the chapter. These descriptions differ among themselves. For some field theorists, especially for those who use phenomenal analysis without a special symbolic apparatus, the person appears to be much the same as in common experience; and the same is true for some social psychologists. The psychoanalyst's 'tragic farce' multiplies the person into a whole cast and concentrates on one aspect of his behaviour: but, for that important aspect, it is close to common experience. In all other psychologies, the person is unrecognizable behind his disguise of figures, formulas, symbols and diagrams. Superficially considered, there are two kinds of psychological theory: literary, corresponding to the plain language generalizations of common experience, and abstract symbolic, corresponding to the generalizations of the sciences.

The argument about the methods and operations of psychology leads on to other possibilities. It is at least not self-evident that the different special methods and operations are alternative and equally permissible ways of setting about the same task. Even less is it self-evident that differences between special methods and the methods of common experience are of this trivial order. But there may be no common task. Prior to differences in operations, there may be differences in the apprehension of the general characteristics of human behaviour.

Differences of this kind are evident with regard to the person's engagement with his environment. It does not need a profound introspective analysis to discover that life is active, turbulent, eventful and tense; nor an exhaustive enumeration to show that it is like this for everyone, in his nature, whatever his circumstances. Everyone strives for mastery over things and everyone is at times at war with other persons and with himself; while equally everyone needs other people and can be at peace with himself only if he goes out to meet them. The scale or scope of activity may vary, down to the limit of the catatonic schizophrenic, whose endless wars and reconciliations are conducted in strict privacy; but the nature of activity is universal. So much for common experience. In special experience, the human drama is at least impersonalized or broken into parts. Thus, in social psychology it would be truer to say that the person depends on an impersonal society than to say that he needs other people as persons. In psychoanalysis the drama is removed from real life to the ghostly stage of the unconscious and in phenomenal analysis it is somewhat attenuated by concentration on the hero to the relative exclusion of the rest of the cast. In the other psychologies, the human drama is not merely reduced, it is ignored.

Much the same is found with the person's history, which is his engagement considered over the longest possible time. In common experience, this has a dramatic articulation, though not necessarily unity, similar to the articulation of the shorter drama of the person's present engagement. One action leads into another with a certain unified development and even inevitability. In psychology little of this appears. It does appear in the work of the more clinically minded phenomenal analysts, though not in that of other field theorists. In psychoanalysis, because of its special interests, there is no real history, but only a tragic repetition of ineffective ritual. The social psychologists are inclined to treat the person's development more as his automatic responses to a changing environment than as a coherent plot. In the other psychologies, again, there is no history.

The case is similar with regard to the causes of the person's behaviour. Common experience allows that the person is the agent of his own becoming; while it may go as far as the vulgar error that his behaviour is free in the sense of unconstrained or even uncaused, at least it does not assert that the person is passive, moved only by external forces. Nor does any psychology assert this, but psychoanalysis comes close to it, as its internalized forces are all of purely external origin; and some social psychology comes even closer. Phenomenal analysis makes reasonable allowance for the person's initiative, but for the other schools of psychology, in which the person is isolated and has no history, the question is naturally irrelevant.

These peculiarities in the general apprehension of human behaviour might be due merely to a specialization of interest in psychology. Thus the general empiricist and the physiological psychologist would ignore the person's environment and history *because* their fields do not include these topics: and so on. But this would be reasonable only if the different psychologies set out to be, not psychology at large, but contiguous and independent technologies within psychology. In so far as their approaches are specialized, the schools do tend to be separate technologies, but they tend equally towards generality. Empirical psychology includes the scientific study of personality, not merely of test measurements, and physiological psychology propounds the laws of learning, not merely of maze-running. Social psychology traces the development and the variations of personality and psychoanalysis in return explains the whole structure of society. It could hardly be otherwise, indeed. However it may be with applied psychology proper (e.g. human engineering), it would be surprising if other psychologies were content with a technical concentration on practical problems, leaving the development of psychology at large to time and chance. The specializations of interest of psychology cannot be so simply explained; and here again it may be profitable to look for determinative prior assumptions.

These are easily found. The psychologist's assumptions about the nature and conditions of valid knowledge may be expected at least to influence his general apprehension of human behaviour as well as his detailed methods of selecting and handling information. The aim of psychology is to be scientific: that is, to substitute exact and demonstrable knowledge for the vague and inarticulate knowledge of common experience. The psychologist must therefore have some ideas on what is and what is not admissible as evidence: and it is these ideas that remain to be examined.

The idea of degrees of knowledge may be taken first. In common experience, knowledge ranges widely from detailed, exact and communicable to fragmentary, vague and incoherent. At the one extreme, the person certainly knows his name, address, age, telephone number, and so on; and he certainly knows and can repeat them exactly. At the other extreme, it may be that the person has an unpleasant feeling of apprehension. He feels quite fit and is certain that he is not suffering from a general bodily malaise; but, however much he thinks about his feeling, he cannot attach it to a specific worry and say of what he is apprehensive. He cannot even describe the feeling very clearly. It feels as if something dreadful is going to happen, or has happened: something physically painful, or terrifying, or embarrassing, or humiliating, he cannot say which. However, he is certain he has the feeling and he is certain of its generally threatening quality: so that for him the feeling ranks as knowledge. If he still feels apprehensive the next day, and can dimly recall two or three similar episodes in the past, or can then tentatively identify the object of his feeling, he will include this memory and this perception as knowledge in their uncertain degree.

How the psychologist treats this range depends on his school. The phenomenal analysts tend to accept the whole range, perhaps without even distinguishing sufficiently between the clear and the unclear. The psychoanalysts are equally willing to accept unclear evidence, providing they can clarify it by interpretation within the framework of their system. Social psychology has been much concerned with the conditions under which knowledge is distorted, false or inadequate, and therefore accepts the range of clarity incidentally in allowing that persons may have some idea, but a very unclear idea, of (for example) the structure of their society. For the other two schools, the empiricists and especially the physiologists, there are no degrees of knowledge: there is only knowledge as it is supposed to be in the sciences, exact and fully communicable, and then ignorance.

The idea of degrees of knowledge involves the subsidiary idea of subjective and objective knowledge. In common experience one assumes that a person's behaviour is intentional in the same sense as one's own, and one then interprets the behaviour (whether an act or, more usually, speech) by attaching it to its perceived intention. If for any reason interpretation is not possible, observed behaviour stands by itself as objective knowledge. In psychology there are three ways of handling this question. The phenomenal analysts, together with some social psychologists, and the psychoanalysts prefer or are at least quite willing to accept behaviour that is open to intentional interpretation; and they make the interpretation. Other social psychologists and some empiricists are prepared to accept interpretable behaviour so long as it is not interpreted: one knows what the person said and can include it in a statistical category, but one does not know what he meant. The rigorously scientific psychologists accept only performances from which the person's intention can hardly be inferred, whether test measurements, as used by the empiricist, or physiological observations.

Another idea which derives from that of degrees of knowledge is that psychological propositions range from strongly to weakly verifiable. In common experience, propositions that are too complex and too speculative to be capable of anything but weak verification are accepted as empirical: one acts on a weakly verified proposition. Most psychologists do this too, but there is a tendency in some schools to test only propositions that are easy to verify or disprove, which largely means testing propositions that are of little generality even if their statistical verification is highly probable. The rigorous requirement that only strongly verifiable propositions should be examined is laid down by some physiological and empirical psychologists but is not uniformly taken into practice.

It may be concluded that differences among psychologies and, even more, differences between psychology and common experience derive firstly from different conceptions of the scientific status of psychology. Here again, it is at the least not self-evident that psychology is or could be a science in the same sense and through the same kind of operations as the natural sciences. It is at the least possible that there are distinctive characteristics, and therefore distinctive laws, for the order of human being in the same way as there are for the distinct orders of physical and animal being.

It seems, indeed, that psychologists may have been a little rash both in disowning their philosophical ancestors, whose ideas on cosmology might save them from a premature acceptance of physicalism, and in snubbing their poor relations in the field of common experience, whose knowledge might help them to avoid a too narrow professionalism. It is certainly not suggested that psychology has been consistently on the wrong path or that it is of no value: on the contrary, its proved value in clarifying, extending and correcting

10

common experience is sufficient demonstration of the soundness of its growth. None the less, it seems necessary that the question of psychology's place in the whole field of experience, and not merely in the special field of the sciences, should be examined in detail. A convenient way of doing this is to reverse the introductory argument and start by considering the nature of evidence, go on to the general characteristics of human behaviour and then consider the technical implications of the more general argument. In conclusion, the social development and determining conditions of psychology will be considered.

FACT AND INTERPRETATION IN PSYCHOLOGY

PERHAPS the simplest way of opening the discussion of the nature and status of evidence in psychology is to consider the distinction between the raw observed fact and the reported interpretation of it. This distinction is not peculiar to psychology. In the sciences, the fact is strictly the instrument reading or the microscopic section described simply as a visual percept, and the report of twenty milliamps or a diseased adrenal cortex is in a sense an interpretation. In history, it is a fact that the Council of Constance condemned Hus in 1415, but to say that this event set the Utraquist movement going is clearly to make an interpretation. The difference between the two cases is instructive. In science, it is simply assumed that experimenters' perceptions agree, so that interpretative reports are accepted from any trained observer. In history, however, agreement among competent workers on the kind of interpretation mentioned may be expected only after long public discussion, if indeed it is reached at all. Of course interpretations of this order are not unlike the general hypotheses of science, which undergo an equally elaborate public examination before they are accepted. But even if the comparison is shifted to this ground, the difference remains. Science can build on a solid ground of agreed interpretation, while the basis of history, if it is not merely a matter of opinion, is always open to re-examination.

The aim of psychology may be to avoid the uncertainties of history and to approximate the exactness of science. Its first step, therefore, is to decide what kinds of information are capable of exact handling and to accept only these. This step will require the examination of the whole apparent range from precise to vague information: that is, from data which are reliable and which can be classified without ambiguity to data of doubtful reliability and uncertain meaning. The most precise information is an instrument reading: megohms, reaction time, force of contraction. Next to this come measurements in the forced choice type of cognitive test (abilities and aptitudes), closely followed by similarly constructed tests of interests, social skills and personality traits. Then there is the observation of behaviour, which leaves some room for disagreement between observers if the behaviour is fairly complex (e.g. who speaks to whom in a group of persons). Following this comes the questionnaire type of interview, in which questions are asked in a fixed order and with a fixed form of words, but the subject replies in his own words; and this leads into the check list type of interview, in which only the areas to be explored are defined. The last and least precise information is that which is gathered in casual conversation or casually overheard.

Now all these ways of getting information are scientifically valid and acceptable so long as they yield data that are capable of objective treatment. This means, first and foremost, data that can be used without anything being read into them. The experimenter must be able to compare records for different persons, or for the same person at different times or under different conditions, without in any way interpreting his data. With some kinds of data, this is easy. A reading of seventeen megohms or 138 milliseconds can only mean the same as an identical reading, even if this identity is interpreted at a later stage of the argument. With some other kinds of data, identity can at least be assumed, as it usually is. Thus two persons have identical scores on a test of intelligence or stenographic aptitude or job interests or introversion if their total scores are the same, however much the patterns of their answers may differ. A similar assumption can be made with observed behaviour, where even a complex case can be simplified by the convention that remarks not addressed to another person by name (for example) will be recorded as addressed to the whole group. The treatment of data from either kind of open interview is not quite so easy, but it can be done if the material is classified by an analysis of content, based on the superficially apparent similarity of responses. This requires the nice distinction among differences in wording of those that are sufficient to constitute a difference in classification from those that are not. Thus the workman who describes his foreman as 'good-oh', his workmates generally as 'dinkum' and his particular mate as 'bonzer' may or may not have the same attitude to all three: and three workmen who use these different words for the one object may or may not be classified together.

In fact, even in this hair-splitting case, one may have to go beyond the superficially apparent similarity of responses and interpret them with reference to the person's intentions. With fairly detailed material, such as the person's report of his habitual behaviour at home or at work, or of his history or his aspirations, the reference to his intentions is almost inevitable. But the difference between this kind of case and the case where no reference is made to the person's intentions must not be exaggerated. The psychologist naturally assumes, in the same way as everyone else, that behaviour is intentional. If his own behaviour were not, he would not be experimenting and if his subject's behaviour were not he would be getting no coherent responses. Where psychologists differ is in their choice of methods for delimiting the person's intentions and controlling them during the experiment.

In the objective measurement situation, whether physical measurements are made or forced choice cognitive tests are used, the person intends only to do what the experimenter tells him to do. The experimenter plays safe by making only this minimal assumption, which is doubtless reasonably made, about his subject's intentions. Whether his data can then be related to ordinary intentional behaviour is not so clear; but this must be put aside for consideration later. This point does not arise, of course, with other procedures which are designed to get evidence of intentional behaviour, but these procedures differ considerably among themselves in the extent to which they delimit the person's intentions in advance. So far as their items refer to deliberate behaviour, inventory type tests of interests, social adjustment or personality traits all invite the subject to express his intentions or habits in a large number of hypothetical situations. Thus he may be asked whether he would prefer visiting the zoo to seeing a football match; whether he takes the lead in discussions, or whether he daydreams frequently. This kind of information is interpreted fact, not plain fact. The construction of the test depends on the decision that identical responses will be treated as having the same reasons: and this decision is an interpretation. On whatever ground of experience, the interpretation is made that there is only one reason for preferring the zoo to football and only one cause of daydreaming: or, if there is variety in these matters, it can be ignored as insignificant. Interview procedures depend on a different and much more open kind of interpretation. Whether the invitation to the person is formal and invariable or open and flexible, he is invited to report his experience (or past intentional behaviour), his habitual behaviour, his opinions, intentions for the future, and so on. Handling this kind of information requires only the assumption that the person's intentions can be inferred from what he says, so that the inference is made afterwards and in the particular case, instead of before and generally.

Wherever the psychologist sets out to investigate something, he starts with a hypothesis. He expects reaction time to change, spatial

14

ability to remain constant, introversion to differ or perception of social class to be determined, under a variety of specified conditions. He expects these events because he has met something like them before, whether in his daily experience or in the course of his professional work. He begins by interpreting the experience of others in relation to his own experience, then he engages in activity with other persons which is designed to test his interpretation, then he either changes his interpretation and tests again, or confirms it and leaves it until new experience broadens it. The sequence of interpretation, test and re-interpretation goes on as long as the person is capable of learning from new experience: in this, the practice of psychology follows life at large. Further, it may now be suggested that somewhere in this universal sequence every kind of psychology is bound to make interpretations which are at least related to the common experience of behaviour, if they are not directly intentional. This is obviously true of the kind of psychology which, as Snygg and Combs [63, p. 11] put it, aims: 'to observe behaviour from the point of view of the individual himself'. It is equally true for the psychologists who measure objectively the person's interests, traits and attitudes, when they go on to draw inferences about the significance of their measurements in the person's daily behaviour. Their initial assumption, discussed above, that identical statements signify identical motives or intentions is an interpretation of behaviour (if it is not merely a blind assumption) that comes before the first and every subsequent investigation in the indefinite sequence. The interpretation of their first results with reference to daily behaviour comes before the second and every subsequent investigation in the sequence. Interpretative reference to common experience as a source of knowledge is therefore inevitable from the second stage of any continuously developed work. It may be doubted whether this reference can really be excluded from the first stage, in which a hypothesis about the relations among purely objective measures is formulated.

With the most objective measures, instrument readings or scores on forced choice cognitive tests, there is less trouble at the first stage. Interests, traits and attitudes may have analogues in common experience, while skin resistance and mechanical comprehension are studied only by the psychologist. In the first stage of his work he will still have to interpret experience before he can formulate a hypothesis: but what he will interpret is exclusively in the professional field, sharply defined in its nature and carefully reported by his colleagues. In the second stage of interpretation, however, he has the same trouble as anyone else. If he wants to relate changes in skin resistance to emotional behaviour in ordinary life, or mechanical comprehension scores to the actual detailed handling of machines, he has to draw on common experience as much as his less scientific colleagues. Of course he does not have to discuss these or any other real life relations. It would be quite logical for the pure empiricist to construct a whole psychology out of behaviour which occurs nowhere but in the laboratory or the test room. However, life seems to break in regardless of scientific intentions, so that not even the hardiest empiricist has tried this consistently.

It may be concluded provisionally that the distinction between fact and interpretation is a logical distinction which is necessary in both analysis and synthesis, but which cannot serve as a criterion for accepting or rejecting evidence. The argument may be taken a stage further by considering the point already made in passing, that interpreting the experience of others means relating it to one's own experience. This also is true, though in somewhat different ways, of every kind of psychology. At one extreme, in handling open interview material, the experimenter may refer the person's behaviour directly to his own experience in order to infer intentions. This is a simple analogical judgement: 'what would I mean if I said that'. It can be referred to past or present experience or to imaginary experience. It is a common, if only an implicit, component of the practical judgements of daily life in all new personal situations (which means practically all situations) and it is probably a component of most of the psychologist's complex judgements of persons. At the other extreme, in handling objective measurements, the experimenter's reference to himself is more limited, but is none the less inevitable if he is to understand what he is doing, which means understanding a problem presented in someone else's behaviour. Now, as Ryle [58, p. 54] puts it: 'Understanding is a part of knowing *how*. The knowledge that is required for understanding intelligent performances of a specific kind is some degree of competence in performances of that kind.' The experimenter may be concerned with deciding how his subjects would perform on a test of abstract verbal ability which is similar to one they have done: or with deciding how to improve the items of an existing test, or how to construct a test. In all these cases he is formulating a hypothesis about a specific performance and in all, especially in the last, he refers to his own experience of and competence in handling items and tests of the kind in question. Some such reference is inevitable, whether he works right through a pool of items or series of tests, noting his judgements as he goes along, or whether he hurriedly selects items that look promising at a quick glance. The quickest glance still refers him to his own experience. Further, this still holds where the innovations he is proposing are less in extent. In the limiting case that he reads an account of an investigation and decides to repeat it, with the same test material,

16

but with different subjects, he has to understand a specific intelligent performance (that of the author), which means deciding what he would have meant if he had written it. Here he may be referring to his past experience, both in his professional training and in his general symbolic learning, rather than his present experience: but refer to his experience he must, however hastily and tacitly.

This again is as true in common experience as it is in the professional experience of the psychologist. Taken together with the universality of interpretation in knowledge, it amounts only to a statement of the general basis of learning. All learning depends on the reflexive interpretation of one's experience together with the experience of others. In social learning, this interpretation is direct, as Mead [45, p. 73] observes: 'When the response of the other person is called out and becomes a stimulus to control his action, then he has the meaning of the other person's act in his own experience.' Ricoeur [56, pp. 13, 14] similarly observes that one knows not merely external facts about someone, but his intentional acts, and that one knows other persons in knowing oneself and oneself in knowing others. Symbolic and perceptual learning, or learning ideas and learning about things, are not so directly dependent on reflexive interpretation in a personal relation simply because some of one's learning of these kinds may be done alone. But only some can be: impersonal learning depends ultimately on personal if it is to be socialized and testable, that is, communicable. Gilson [26, p. 296] [1] puts the general case thus: 'La perception sensible est donc l'échange vital qui se produit sans cesse entre des êtres intelligents et des choses réellement existantes. Elle est, en fait, le point de rencontre de deux actes distincts d'exister.'

It follows that communication between persons necessarily refers to the experience of both persons, so that the distinction between facts that refer only to the experience of the person reporting them and subjective interpretations of these facts is, in general, false. Even the most exact communication is reflexive. If the histology demonstrator says to the students: 'Look for the star-shaped cells with purple-stained nuclei', he is not only pointing to the student's potential or future experience, he is also pointing to his own experience. What he is saying is: 'My perception of this preparation is as I have described it on the basis of my previous perceptual and symbolic learning, and if you look at the same preparation you will see something that you may or may not describe in the same way.' Further, even rudimentary communication is in a sense reflexive.

---

[1] 'Sensory perception, then, is the living exchange which incessantly takes place between intelligent beings and things that really exist. It is, in fact, the meeting place of two distinct acts of existing.'

The mere gesture of handing a completed test to the tester can hardly imply anything beyond itself. But in so far as the person thereby publicly accepts his fate, he is pointing to the experimenter's future experience in marking the test and perhaps to his past experience in constructing it, as well as to his own experience in doing it. Of course in this case the experience of each person is something that the other person can hardly even imagine, let alone know exactly: but this means only that communication, while it is always reflexive in principle, is not effective unless the parties are on common ground, and this is already implied in the first example. In principle, then, any communicable event ranks as knowledge which psychology can accept, but in practice there are sharp limitations on what can be communicated at all, let alone communicated exactly.

THE DEGREES OF KNOWLEDGE

Limitations in the person's knowledge of himself may be considered first. Strictly, he knows only his infinitesimal and continually changing present. The old objection to introspection, that it is really retrospection, may be accepted, but it has little force: the distinction is at the most between certain and highly probable knowledge. One might add to this that, if the distinction is pressed, certain knowledge recedes to infinity, leaving only knowledge that ranges from high to low probability. However, it must be allowed that some events are outside this range altogether. Many of the more trivial events of the present and even more of the past are swept away and lost in the stream. No man can be expected to say for certain whether or not he blew his nose two years ago exactly, or even five minutes ago. The person, then, knows his important activities in the present and to a less extent in the past: but this knowledge too is limited. It is to be expected that under most conditions the person will not know, or will very insufficiently know, his defence mechanisms or his irrational ways of relating his perceptions to his needs. Following Ichheiser's suggestions, [29, Ch. 4], one could include under this head not only the well-known pathological mechanisms, such as projection and repression, but also the person's learnt ways of making personal and social judgements. The more these judgements are rigid, stereotyped and dependent on limited insight, the less likely is the person to know it. If knowledge of the present is so limited, knowledge of the past must be even more limited. Some traumatic memories are actively and completely repressed and others may appear in a form that is remotely derived from the original experience by the working of defence mechanisms at various levels.

Important memories that are not traumatic may be considerably condensed and reorganized as time goes on and some, as Cameron suggests [7, p. 136], may never be fully formed because they are of events that happened too early to be verbalized.

At this point a second set of limitations appears. The person's knowledge of himself may be limited, but it is all equally knowledge in the sense that it is all equally communicable. This is true only if one takes communicability as a distinctive criterion of knowledge: but it may be that one knows more than one can communicate. To say this is not to assert a doctrine of the mysterious faculty of intuition: it is merely to point to the common experience that one sometimes has ideas and feelings that are hard to put into words. As Collingwood [12, p. 200] says, we know our thoughts obscurely before we express them. Whether or not the experience is universal, it is not remarkable, for if all of the person's ideas and feelings are to be capable of clear verbalization, he would have to have a command of language at least equal to that of all the makers of his language together. In fact, some ideas and feelings may need elaboration by further experience, or repeated attempts at verbalization, or both, before they can be put into a form of words that satisfies the person. Whether the obscurely or doubtfully communicable can rank as knowledge in any degree may be questioned: and the answer is to consider how it arises. Firstly, it may be expected that complex matter will be hard to communicate. Under this head one would include any generalization which is at the limit of the person's capacity for intellectual synthesis; generalizations about his main drives and goals or about the major features of the whole course of his life. One would include here also experience which does not yet fit in with the person's language uses because there is not yet enough of it: for example, the foreman knows that there is something he does not quite like about his new boss or his new charge hand, but he cannot put his finger on it. The person would usually regard both these kinds of knowledge as fairly certain and important, at least to him, so that there is no obvious case for ruling them out.

Secondly, it may be expected that persons will differ considerably in their capacity for communication. The experience of early childhood cannot be verbalized, unless one accepts the retrospective interpretation of the patient under psychoanalysis as a direct memory. Much older children verbalize experience less readily than do adults. Differences due to innate intelligence may be expected and differences due to general verbal sophistication will be considerable. The story of the psychiatrist who used to ask his working class outpatients what was their ideal in life, and who was surprised that the usual answer was a blank look, may be untrue. But psychologists have certainly found it easier to work with middle class, and especially undergraduate, subjects, who can at least attempt to answer such a question. Besides this, there may even be differences due to special verbal competence. Especially when the purpose of communication is to point to an obscurely or doubtfully known experience, the poet's use of metaphors, new meanings and improvisations may be more relevant, as Collingwood [12, p. 214] suggests it is for the parallel purpose in philosophy, than the scientist's supposedly univocal language. It must be allowed, of course, that these limitations of expression are closely related to the limitations of the person's knowledge of himself. Communication which strains the person's capacity for expression and the general capacity of his language to the utmost would usually be communication of the obscurely known, for the person knows clearly only what he can express in language. However, whether one says that there are experiences which can hardly be expressed because they can hardly be known or that there are experiences that can hardly be known because they can hardly be expressed, the conclusion is the same: so far as any expression is possible, it ranks as knowledge in some degree.

So far the limitations of what the person can know of himself and what he can tell the psychologist have been considered. It remains to be considered whether there are any limitations of the psychologist's understanding. Where understanding is not required, there is of course no problem. If the psychologist is interested only in external measurements and not in intentional acts, then he knows them as accurately as he knows any ordinary percept. But if his objective measurements are derived from intentional acts, interpreted generally and before the event, and especially if he is directly concerned with intentional acts, the case is different. It has already been argued that, because of the reflexive nature of communication, the intentional interpretation that he is bound to make whether or not he realizes it depends on some reference to analogies in his own experience: and this immediately introduces limitations.

The psychologist has some analogous experience in the course of his professional work, in that he can refer back to similar cases. This experience is obviously limited, both in extent and in variety, for not even the busiest psychologist can know professionally more than a few persons and he would usually know them in a limited context only. Besides this, such experience is limited in its nature. It is vicarious or indirect experience of the experience of others, not a direct analogue of their behaviour. The most it can do is to help the psychologist construct imaginary experience which is analogous to that of his subjects. If a psychologist of schizoid character, for example, hears about and sees the compulsive's detailed, unvarying and fastidious routine for his dressing and personal toilet, often enough, he will be better able to imagine himself doing such things and to understand why people do them, even if his routine is characteristically careless. Similarly, if he often enough hears about and sees the hysteroid's habit of rejecting tasks with indifference or contempt as soon as they become difficult, he will be better able to imagine himself doing this even though his own work habits are tenacious to the point of rigidity. None the less, he does not have the compulsive's or the hysteroid's experience and cannot have it unless he wants it as they do; that is, unless he is a compulsive or a hysteroid. The most he can do is to imagine the experience: and this is obviously a very limited basis for making analogical interpretations or intention.

The psychologist can, of course, refer to his own real experience, either present or past, whenever it appears to be analogous and, superficially considered, this will cover a wide range of common behaviour. Everyone dresses, eats and goes to bed; most persons marry and bring up children; many persons go to work; and so on. However, people do not necessarily do these things in the same way. A little attention to the individuality of common experience will compel an interpretation of its uncommon elements and will lead the psychologist directly back to relying in some degree on constructed imaginary experience. The psychologist's self-reference in making an analogical judgement will usually be to a compound of his own real ordinary experience interpreted in the light of the imaginary experiences derived from his professional experience. His construction of the person's point of view may have a solid basis in both ordinary and professional experience, but it is a complex and elaborate construction and by no means an immediate percept. It follows that the psychologist's reflexive judgements will be limited by his knowledge of himself in some of the ways that his subjects' reports are limited. The psychologist's intelligence, general education and special training should give him an advantage over his subject, especially in his handling of the more complex and obscure kinds of knowledge. Beyond this, there will still be plenty that he cannot know exactly because in its nature it is not accessible to full analysis or because of various distortions of his perception of himself of which he is unaware. Training in psychology may make him aware of the ideological elements in his self-perception and these will then no longer be distortions, for if he is aware of them he can to some extent discount them in seeing the other's point of view. The defence mechanisms that partly determine his self-perception are not so easily managed; merely being aware of these may be easy to achieve but by no means guarantees that they will not be used.

The last limitation that needs to be considered is that even where the psychologist's knowledge depends on real experience similar to that of his subject, this experience is only similar, not identical. It cannot be identical, for everyone knows directly only himself in the world, which is his private world, as he perceives it. Of course there is no need to exaggerate the privacy of the person's knowledge of himself. In arguing against the doctrine of privileged access, Ryle [58, p. 172] observes: 'The ascertainment of a person's mental capacities and propensities is an inductive process, an induction to law-like propositions from observed actions and reactions.' Thus there is no behaviour which is inaccessible in principle to inductive (or analogical) inference. On the other hand, there is no need to exaggerate the accessibility of other persons' experience. Much of this may be inaccessible in practice, or accessible only in some degree, to inductive inference. Thus when Stevens [66, p. 27] asserts that: 'Not even psychology knows anything about private experience, because an operation for penetrating privacy is self-contradictory', he goes too far. If all other limitations were removed, the limitation would remain that similar experience is not identical. This may be of no practical importance with the experience of colour discrimination or of arithmetical addition, but there are many experiences of importance to the psychologist as well as to his subject which are by no means as simple as this.

The general conclusion is that psychology has a range of degrees of knowledge. There is the knowledge of bare fact, where the experimenter can read the instrument as accurately as any other experimenter and need do nothing beyond that, for he cannot interpret the subject's intentions. At the other extreme, there is the experience which the person hardly knows and must struggle to express in words and which the experimenter, in making a reflexive interpretation of the person's experience, can hardly imagine, let alone relate to his own real experience. But this, if it is much less exact than the instrument reading, is still knowledge in its degree; for neither party is completely ignorant of the matter of communication and either may find his knowledge sufficient to act on. It can be said, indeed, that knowledge ranges continuously in the degree of its exactness: for the hardiest empiricist would surely accept the simplest interpretations of intention as being as accurate as his instrument readings. The practical question is only where in the continuous range should the psychologist draw the line and declare that beyond it is knowledge too vague to be used. One answer to this is to exclude all intentional acts and to confine psychology as MacMurray [42, p. 248] puts it, to investigating 'the means of intentional actions'. Whether the objective measurements that this answer depends on can claim a superior status is a question that must be considered in the next chapter. Here it is sufficient to observe that if intentional acts are excluded from the body of knowledge, psychology abandons its claim to deal directly with ordinary behaviour at all; and it is not self-evident that this is necessary or desirable. Further, if some intentional acts are admitted, there is no ground for excluding others, however obscurely known they may be. Obscure knowledge, which is often knowledge of centrally important behaviour, may be provisional and speculative but it is neither mysterious nor totally unreliable. It is, indeed, prominent in the knowledge on which persons do act, quite confidently and often quite successfully, in the course of their daily lives. If the psychologist is to exclude it, and even more if he is to exclude all knowledge of intentional acts, he is bound to do violence to himself as a person. He may accept knowing less than any ordinary person does about others, both in his professional work and in his daily life, being rigorously objective throughout. In this case he accepts being less than a person. Or he may prefer to be rigorously scientific in his work and ordinarily human elsewhere, in which case he is two incompatible persons.

It seems much simpler to abandon the artificial distinction between science and life and to use the whole of one's evidence, judgement, experience and insight as wholeheartedly in one's work as one does in one's life. The rather neglected empirical questions of the nature and conditions of sound judgement and so on then become important: but these too must be deferred.

THE INSUFFICIENCY OF THE
OBJECTIVE

THE fascinating possibility that one could make a sufficient study of the person by treating him as an object must now be considered. The psychologist may decide to ignore the fact that the object is a person, co-ordinate with him and, like him, prone to intentional behaviour; and to study this object, as far as possible, by doing only such things to it as he could do to any other living object. There are several kinds of thing that he can do. Firstly, he may rely on test measurements and other measurements of the person's behaviour. This may not be an entirely objective procedure, for the use of tests of attitudes, interests and traits with items requiring the expression of intentional behaviour depends on interpretation, at least during the construction of the test. This qualification is of little practical importance, however, so long as the use of the results is rigorously empirical; that is, so long as scores on tests and scales are used for statistical but not for interpretative prediction. The qualification hardly applies to tests with items that do not tap ordinary behaviour and does not apply to the measurement of eye blinks, rate of breathing and so on. Procedures of this kind, unless they are used solely for their own sake, depend on the assumption that findings derived only remotely or not all from ordinary behaviour can be transferred to ordinary behaviour. As this is usually more complex than the behaviour studied, the transfer usually requires a sort of axiom in addition. It is assumed, for example, that scores on social attitude scales add to give the person's motives in social behaviour; or that scores on tests of ability add to give his performance in an examination or in his work; or that measurements of vascular and respiratory changes add to give his emotional state. These assumptions are necessary if the psychology of objective measurement aims to be psychology at large; but they are not self-evident and must therefore be examined in due course.

The second objective procedure is to experiment on animals. This is usually done for its own sake and its popularity may be due to its ease: animals are cheap and expendable and can be treated with less respect than persons. However, perhaps because of its popularity, the method is sometimes put forward as relevant to psychology at large in that it gives indirect evidence on human behaviour. Thus findings about animal learning may be transferred almost as they stand to human learning, though few psychologists do this explicitly. Some others give the impression that they expect animal psychology to provide the first part of a developing series of behaviour which can be extrapolated to include human behaviour. The common assumption is, at the least, that there are useful analogies between animal and human behaviour, and hence some possibility of transferring findings. This assumption is made only incidentally, for animal psychologists are usually little concerned with human behaviour; but, as it is made, it too must be examined in due course.

The last and most radical objective procedure is the exclusive use of observations of the nervous system, especially of the brain. In the present state of experimental psychology it is a hypothetical rather than an actual procedure, for the observation of cortical potential waves by means of the electroencephalograph is almost the practical limit in this field. However, cerebral physiology is developing rapidly and the promise is sometimes made, or implied, that it is only a matter of time before the person's inmost behaviour, his thoughts and emotions as well as his perceptions and speech, will be directly observable on the appropriate instruments. The assumption here is that a diagram of potential sequences in a cortical circuit points to the same event as does the person's report of the solution to an arithmetical problem, for example. This is an assumption, not of addition or transfer or analogy, but of equivalence or identity. If it is true, it might make the other objective procedures, let alone the ordinary study of behaviour, simply unnecessary; which is sufficient ground for considering it first.

THE IRRELEVANCE OF PHYSIOLOGY

The first point that must be taken is that this assumption is not at present an empirical proposition: it cannot be tested against the facts of cerebral physiology because these facts are too scanty to offer any but the weakest support or refutation. It is an assumption about the venerable body-mind problem, but what it does is to assert rather than to argue a solution. This may be demonstrated by a brief consideration of some recent views on this problem.

A clear and elaborate case is put by Ryle [58], who argues at length that the problem is spurious. The 'dogma of the ghost in the machine' inserts an unknowable and mysterious agent as the controller of the person on the mistaken view that the person and his mind are separate entities. If one takes the person to be a coherent and self-controlling system, the agent, or ghost, is simply dispensed with. This view so neatly removes the considerable difficulties of the classical dualistic theories, parallelism and interactionism, that one would expect it to be held, if only implicitly, by other workers in the field. But this is not so. Mead's interest in the problem [45, p. 187] is limited to a remark which is most easily read in an interactionist sense: 'The legitimate basis of distinction between mind and body is between the social patterns and the patterns of the organism itself.' The general texts in psychology tend to ignore the body-mind problem, by giving detailed accounts of bodily and mental functions without discussing the relation between the two. Nor are the physiologists more inclined to monism. Hebb [27, Introduction] is at least disinclined definitely to reject interactionism and Tinbergen [68, p. 206] rather suggests a dualistic division between the objective facts of neurology and the subjective and only partly corresponding facts of experience. The dualistic view is openly stated by Eccles [19, Ch. 8], who answers Ryle's case by observing that the brain is a small and very sensitive machine that could be worked by a mere whisper of a ghost, such as the experience of telepathy points to.

The status of the initial assumption that cortical events and events in experience are equivalent or identical can now be more clearly seen. It is in line with Ryle's philosophical case but does not meet it as Ryle does not consider the implications of his view for cerebral physiology. The assumption may or may not be in line with the facts of psychology and physiology; one cannot say, because the psychologists and physiologists have not considered it. There is thus a gap in the argument: nobody seems to have considered just what the identity of cortical events and ordinary experience would mean. Obviously this must be considered, however speculatively, before the possible consequences of this identity in the practice of psychology can be considered.

The simplest way of considering this hypothetical identity is to state that the cortical event and the person's experience are not two distinct events but only two distinct ways of perceiving the same event. The person, as Collingwood [13, Ch. 2] says, may be studied as body or as mind, but he is one person studied in two different ways. For example, the person says to the experimenter: 'I see red.' This event is a sequence of five separate physical systems, each of which can be traced in detail. Light waves reflected from a red object into the person's eyes are followed by systematic potential changes in the retinae, occipital cortex, association areas, motor areas and nerves of the larynx. The last of these changes is followed by contractions of the muscles of the larynx, these are followed by sound waves, and these by systematic potential changes in the experimenter's cochleae, auditory areas and association areas. This is the ordinary case, in which the person reports his experience and the experimenter hears his report. Given a hypothetical apparatus the experimenter could trace the person's neural event, from retinae through to association areas. If he did this, his neural event (or experience) would be quite different. He would see some kind of instrument reading or record, instead of hearing a report, and the neural event would then proceed from his retinae through the occipital cortex instead of from his cochleae through the auditory areas. The same applies to the subject. He can hear himself making a report or, given the apparatus, he can see the recording of the neural event. In these two cases his secondary neural events, in knowing his own experience, are again distinct. In the one case the secondary event proceeds from his cochleae through the auditory areas, in the other case from his retinae through the occipital cortex. But the subject's initial event or perception is one and the same neural event, proceeding from retinae through to association areas, however he and the experimenter apprehend it: it *is* the subject seeing red.

If it can be worked out further, this would seem to be an attractive idea. It would avoid the notorious logical difficulties of any dualistic view and it would have practical advantages in psychology. It would no longer be necessary to distinguish mental, physical and mixed disorders (or functional, organic and psychosomatic) by attempting the impossible task of drawing a fine line between body and mind. Hysterical and toxic gastritis, for example, would be distinguished by their causal sequences, the one starting with cerebral events and the other with the ingestion of a poison. Further, the distinctions between conscious and unconscious behaviour, and perhaps among semi-conscious, sub-conscious and pre-conscious behaviour as well, should be much easier to handle. It may be noted, too, that the assumption of the identity of the neural event with experience fully allows for the unique status of man and could even be said to put the difference between man and animals exactly where it belongs. Notwithstanding the views of some biologists, the person does not behave like an animal only rather more so: in animal society, if it is properly called society, there is no analogue to communication in the human sense. In spite of the firm beliefs of those persons who substitute pets for children, no animal has ever behaved even remotely like a person in mastering things, in talking or (one must presume) in thinking. Between man and animals, differences of kind in behaviour are gross and obvious and cannot be explained away. But exactly the same is true of the differences in brain structure between man and the apes, let alone between man and lower animals. However, there is no need to argue the case for physiological monism, the detailed consideration of which would be out of place here. The point at issue is the status or relevance of physiological evidence of behaviour and, as the monistic view may be presumed to give this evidence maximum status, it will be sufficient to trace what the consequences would be if this view were true.

In the first place, a hypothetical classification of behaviour according to its complexity may be suggested. The most complex behaviour, which is roughly equivalent to conscious behaviour, is more or less specific events in the association areas that fire or could fire specific events in the motor areas, which then operate the muscles of the larynx, throat, tongue, etc., to issue in speech. The last phase in this sequence is necessarily specific: under normal conditions one either speaks clearly or not at all. It must be presumed that the events of the phase before, in the motor areas, are equally specific. But this need not hold for the first phase, events in the association areas. From the subject's point of view, some experiences may be more easily reported in a precise form of words, so that one might suppose that some sensations, ideas and memories are specific association area events while kinaesthetic sensations and emotions, for example, are less specific events.

A more important point is that the possibility, not the fact, of verbal report is taken as a rough definition of conscious behaviour. From the subject's point of view, it is obvious that much experience which could be verbally reported is not. The person cannot attend to two things at once, so that he cannot report that he has a headache while he is reporting an idea, and vice versa. He may have an idea that he does not wish to report, or which he cannot report because he is alone; and, while this kind of idea may get as far as subvocal speech (or minimal stimulation of the speech muscles), there is no need to suppose that it must. Lastly, there are repressed memories which the subject cannot report except under special conditions. It is assumed that the unreported ideas and sensations are, and the repressed events were, conscious behaviour. Now presumably this scheme can be reproduced from the experimenter's point of view. This is easily done if one supposes that specific events in the association areas may occur simultaneously and may combine or may interfere with each other in various ways. Thus a specific event which by itself would fire the next event in the sequence, in the motor areas, may be interfered with or suppressed by another of exactly the same order: which would be the case that two simple events cannot be reported simultaneously. If the interfering event corresponds to a temporary but general disposition, one has the case that the person does not wish to report; and if it is a permanently firing inhibitory circuit, one has the case of repression.

The two aspects of unconscious behaviour can be traced similarly, though they are not so obviously distinct. From the subject's point of view, unconscious behaviour is what his body does without his knowing it, except indirectly from its effects. Thus he does not know his glandular or muscular changes, but does know that he feels tense or that he is picking up a hammer. He does not know any of the low level neural events that bypass the association areas, such as his postural reflexes; but he does know their effects, such as that he is sitting or walking. He does not know the last details of even his simple thinking, though he certainly knows the results: for example, he knows the answer to an intelligence test question without always being able to say exactly how he reached the answer. Lastly, he may not know all of his more complex thinking. It is a common experience that the solution to a problem may emerge suddenly, hours or even days after one thinks one has stopped thinking of it.

The experimenter can analyse and clarify all these implicit sequences of behaviour. The subject feels tense because his blood pressure has risen, because his adrenal glands have discharged; and he has picked up the hammer because his arm muscles have worked, and so on. With neural events, and especially with cerebral events, the experimenter must depend on supposition. He can assume, for example, that there are events in the association areas which are not large or complex enough to fire specific motor systems, even when there is no interference. These events would be the inaccessible sub-processes of problem solving, for example. Similarly, there may be quite complex events in the association areas that are not specific enough to fire motor events even when there is no interference. These events would be the thoughts that do not emerge in conscious behaviour till they have been elaborated; and many, as Hebb [27, p. 133] suggests, may never emerge at all.

The speculative account of how the person's experience would look to the experimenter who sees it, as it were, indirectly instead of receiving it directly, is now complete. It must be assumed that the experimenter can actually do this; that he possesses an apparatus which will enable him to trace the exact neural paths and potential sequences of, for example, the solution of a geometrical problem. It remains to be considered what the experimenter will gain by using this apparatus.

In real life situations his apparatus will be useless for obvious practical reasons. In the laboratory, where large machines may be handled conveniently, the use of apparatus would be very uneconomical for the study of conscious behaviour. Any behaviour which can be reported, or observed without the use of apparatus, is obviously much more easily studied in the usual way. The same would be true just beyond the limits of the reportable, for comparative experiments (e.g. on problem solving) often enable firm conclusions about sub-processes to be drawn. In the greater part of the whole field of psychology, then, including all conscious behaviour and also behaviour distorted by repressions and including behaviour in constructed as well as real life situations, physiological evidence has nothing to add to the evidence of ordinary phenomenal analysis. It can add nothing for, on the hypothesis which gives it maximum status, it is merely an alternative, elaborately indirect, way of looking at the same events. This conclusion is no more remarkable than the suggestion that one can see one's face more easily, if no more clearly, in a mirror than in a complicated arrangement of prisms and lenses that goes round the house and back again.

None the less, physiological evidence has its place. It might be expected to add precision to the study of truly unconscious behaviour. Behaviour which is unconscious in the sense of being repressed is a special case of conscious behaviour and is irrelevant here, though Tinbergen [68, p. 208] seems to think that 'introspection' is in its nature incapable of revealing the repressed. It is in the study of behaviour which is in its nature incapable of verbal report that the physiological method would be useful. Its field of application would include low level behaviour, such as simple reflexes and muscular and glandular events, though many of these can be either directly observed or unambiguously inferred from observed events. The more important part of the physiological field would be cerebral events which are not large or specific enough to be reportable. The function of physiology, that is to say, is to add precision to the phenomenal study of behaviour by the detailed analysis of events below the phenomenal level.

As the whole account of what physiology might do is necessarily speculative, it is impossible to say just how important this clarification by detailed analysis would be. Time may show that. However, it may be said that detailed analysis would presumably be confined to its own level and would not be able to substitute for phenomenal analysis, as it were by adding sub-processes to make reportable events. This also cannot be firmly asserted in advance of the evidence, but analogies with the sciences suggest that it would be true. The chemist knows the properties of carbon, hydrogen and chlorine but he cannot add them to give the properties of chloroform: he has to study this by itself if he wants to know its properties. Further, if he knows the properties of silicon and silico-chloroform, he may be able to explain the differences found when silicon is substituted for carbon: but he has to know both sets of properties first. The physiologist, again, knows the properties of the heart as a working organ and he may be able to explain them by reference to the properties of the isolated nerve fibre, ordinary heart muscle fibre and pacemaker nodes; but to do this he must study both sets of properties separately; he cannot infer the working of the organ from the properties of its isolated parts.

It is never safe to press an argument by analogy but, so far as this argument can be trusted, it suggests that the particular form of the addition axiom which might be proposed by the physiologist in vindication of the superior status of his evidence should not be accepted until it is tested empirically. The probability then remains that the physiological method cannot in its nature be more than a minor accessory to the phenomenal study of behaviour.

THE INSUFFICIENCY OF ARTIFICIAL BEHAVIOUR

It is now possible to return to the other objective procedures, the use of results obtained with animals and of objective test measurements. Both of these require some kind of assumption or axiom about the transfer or addition of results in order to uphold their claims to superior status. The assumptions actually made are by no means clear but those that would be sufficient can be examined in the light of the available evidence.

In the animal field, nobody is so rash as to claim that results can be transferred generally to human behaviour. However, most workers suggest occasional particular transfers of findings, while they may not be very clear on the basis of these transfers. The general position may be illustrated by Skinner's report [62] of a long series of experiments on rats. He chose the white rat because it is 'an organism as similar to man as is consistent with experimental convenience and control' [62, p. 47]. None the less, his aim was to study rats directly, not persons indirectly, and he makes very few suggestions for the application of his findings to human behaviour. He concludes, however [62, p. 442]:

'We can neither assert nor deny discontinuity between the human and subhuman fields so long as we know so little about either. If, nevertheless, the author of a book of this sort is expected to hazard a guess publicly, I may say that the only differences I expect to see revealed between the behaviour of rat and man (aside from enormous differences of complexity) lie in the field of verbal behaviour.'

This seems to be a quaint way of saying that man is quite like the white rat, except that he is very different in those kinds of behaviour that depend on the use or understanding of language. As this includes most human behaviour, it would appear that discontinuity is asserted. It may be that, if a man were kept in a cage and trained to do circus tricks in order to get his food, he would behave rather like a white rat. But if the similarity expected is between the rat in the cage and the man in the world, one can only say that the whole weight of human experience, though perhaps not that of the psychologist's professional experience, is against the expectation. In any case, as Skinner observes, the expectation is no substitute for evidence. One cannot know how like a rat the person is until one has studied both, so that, unless there is some special interest in answering just this question, it would be cheaper and quicker simply to study man.

It may be as well to make it clear that no objection is advanced against the study of animal psychology in itself. The laws of rat or monkey behaviour are as legitimate as any and, if it is found from parallel experiments that the same laws hold for persons, then the general law including the different species is quite legitimate. What is not legitimate is the transfer to human behaviour of findings derived from experiments on animals when parallel experiments on persons have not been done. While Skinner expressly excludes this transfer, his choice of the white rat because it is 'similar to man' rather suggests the same confusion as is found in many elementary psychology texts, in which the results of animal experiments (e.g. on learning and motivation) are presented in indiscriminate combination with findings derived from persons, regardless of whether or not the animal experiments have been repeated with persons. This loose habit of thought or presentation does not oblige the student to assume that results derived from animal experiments only can be transferred to persons, but it certainly invites him to make the transfer. It is this transfer only which is illegitimate. The simultaneous study of animal and human behaviour may be profitable, but the sole study of the former cannot stand for the direct study of the latter. The conclusion, then, is that animal psychology, whatever its merits as a specialization may be, is irrelevant to psychology at large.

Objective test measurements are easier to discuss because there is some direct experimental evidence about their summation or transferability, though again the addition axiom is never clearly stated.

Particular claims of transferability, however, are made over a wide range. Some social psychologists seem to assume that social attitude scales directly measure the person's effective motivation in social behaviour, though others, such as Krech and Crutchfield [36, Ch. 7], see difficulties in making this transfer. Transferability is more clearly implied in selection testing generally, where measured or rated success on a job is predicted by the addition of scores on psychomotor or cognitive tests, or by some combination of results from these and from situational tests. The clearest claims are within the field of objective test measurement, when psychomotor tests are used to predict job performance under laboratory conditions or cognitive tests are used to predict examination results.

It is the more definite assumptions of the addition axiom that are not supported by the evidence. The results of selection testing are of great practical use but, in the best case, they leave a sufficient margin of unpredicted behaviour to show that any performance in a real job is by no means the simple sum of elementary motor or intellectual capacities. The same is found within the test field itself. Even when the criterion of job performance is itself an exact psychophysical measurement, elementary or analytic psychomotor tests predict it poorly: and cognitive tests do not predict examination results very well, especially at the higher levels. This is often said to be because the criteria are unreliable. But this can hardly be alleged of the most carefully handled job criteria, nor of so-called objective type examinations. It may be noted that the results of these latter are much better predicted by tests which closely resemble them than are the results of essay type examinations. Further, performance in various semi-skilled jobs is much better predicted by tests that are closely analogous to the work task than by tests that analyse it into separate elements. These findings rather suggest that not unreliability, but lack of similarity between predictors and predicted, and especially the analysis of the latter into supposedly additive parts, is the ground of poor results. The evidence suggests, in fact, that where objective test measurements fail to predict equally objective criterion measurements, this is because the criterion is more than, or other than, the simple sum of a number of elementary test abilities or capacities. The suggestion may be generalized to the poor prediction of real life behaviour, though here it is supported by positive evidence only in some cases of job selection. The discussion of the addition axiom must be left at that (except for further references in the more detailed discussion of psychological methods), because of the insufficiency of the evidence. It may be noted, however, that this axiom is not self-evidently plausible. It is a matter of ordinary experience that the pattern of walking, for

33

example, is not learnt by the separate practice of successive movements; or that painting a house is more than the sum of colour discrimination and manual dexterity; or that understanding one's children requires more than averaging one's information about them.

In concluding this discussion, it may be noted that the difficulties of the addition axiom can be avoided by simply making test measurements stand for real behaviour. This is the effect of Eysenck's scientific method of studying personality, which begins [21, p. 3] by proposing to argue: 'from one item of behaviour to another'. It appears, however, that only behaviour in laboratory tests is to be admitted: what the person does, including what he says he does, in real life is not behaviour. The consequence is that neuroticism and psychoticism are defined with scrupulous statistical care in terms of factorial scores on a large number of tests: but neither is directly related to ordinary behaviour. There is no assumption of addition from test to symptom or from the laboratory to the person's work or home, for the person's ordinary life is simply not mentioned. The assumption appears to be that mental disorder can be more reliably diagnosed by the addition of test measurements than by a psychiatrist's interview, or by the patient's own opinion of his condition. That may be so: but it does not follow that the test diagnosis is more reliable than would be a diagnosis made from a similarly exact and detailed analysis of the patient's observed and reported behaviour in his normal environment. As it is this behaviour and not his behaviour in the test room which has to be understood before it can be modified by treatment, there would seem to be no point in the substitution of test measurements for an analysis of ordinary behaviour unless a close equivalence between the two can be assumed. But this assumption is as unwarranted as any other assumption of transferability or addition until it is demonstrated in the particular case. Finally, on the ground of general experience, it is no more likely to be true than is any other such assumption. Neuroticism may be a dimension in a factorial hyperspace but neurosis occurs in the real world.

A general conclusion may be stated briefly. If objective methods of any kind are to be given preference over the intentional analysis of ordinary experience, it can only be because their data are as relevant to the purposes and problems of psychology generally, and are also more exact. The latter may be conceded, though the difference of degree in exactness does not give the objective methods an exclusive right to the name. Except in the special and highly speculative case of physiological observation as an uneconomical way of making direct observations indirectly, equal relevance cannot be taken as established, for all other cases depend on some kind of unproved generalization about the transferability of findings. This may be that cortical sub-processes can be added to give conscious events, or that test results can be added to give real life performances or that findings from animal behaviour can be transferred to man. The common element is the supposition that the simple can be inflated into the complex, or the small magnified into the large. Now all three generalizations are empirical propositions. It may not matter that two at least, which are within the field of common experience, seem unlikely in the light of common experience, though that is by no means to be disregarded as evidence. It does matter that what special evidence there is shows that the generalization about test results must be taken with the greatest reserve. Lastly, it matters most of all that all three generalizations, empirical as they are and therefore capable of systematic test, tend to be tacitly assumed more often than they are stated, and to be stated more often than they are tested. There seems to be little point in staking the future of psychology on general propositions about the nature of evidence which are unlikely, largely untested and suspect where they have been tested.

EMPIRICISM AND EXPERIENCE

THE argument so far has concerned the general nature and limitations of knowledge in psychology and from it two incompatible conclusions can be drawn. The psychologist, accepting his co-ordinate relation with his subject, can accept the fact that the greater part of his knowledge is interpretative and inexact and can develop his work, as far as possible, on the ground of common experience, in deliberate preference to the special experience of the laboratory. On the other hand, even if he agrees that the greater part of his knowledge is the inexact knowledge of common experience and that the remainder is doubtfully relevant to this experience, he may still prefer the rigorous methods of the laboratory. For the aim of psychology is to be a science and, in whatever sense it may become a body of exact knowledge, it can do so only if it includes empirical propositions and no others. From simple propositions that are capable of experimental test more complex propositions can be built up until something like a coherent body of generalizations is achieved. There is no alternative to this procedure: a science can be established only by working from the small to the large or from the parts to the whole.

It may be doubted whether this hypothetical view would be supported by the history of science. Chemistry and physics, for example, began with compounds and with visible energy changes respectively, and took a long time to proceed to molecules and parts of atoms. Biology and physiology began with the description and comparison of structures and with the functions of organs, respectively, and moved on to intra-cellular chemistry in due course. However, an analogy is to be trusted even less when it appears to work both ways than when it gives only one conclusion. The real point to be considered about the scientific status of psychology is what is meant by empirical propositions.

An empirical proposition is one that can be tested in experience.

This distinguishes it from the logical proposition, which is a definition, but this statement is too vague to be itself a definition unless one amplifies the meaning both of testing and of experience. The most rigorous condition for testing would be that anyone should be able to do it easily; and for experience, that a single test should conclusively prove or disprove the proposition. If these conditions were insisted on, very few propositions could be called empirical or verifiable. The condition that the test should be conclusive would exclude all but propositions about single events; for, as Ayer observes [2, p. 9], all other propositions are hypotheses that are under continual test by experience. The probability of an inductive generalization rises as it is found to hold in more and more cases but reaches unity only with complete enumeration. Enumeration cannot be certainly known to be complete unless the proposition is restricted to a single case; that is, unless there is no attempt to generalize beyond the limits in time or number of the instance observed, whether this is a simple or a repeated instance. The other conditions are equally restrictive. That anyone should be able to test the proposition would rule out as unverifiable all propositions the testing of which requires special training. Of course, this requirement is usually understood to mean anyone with the appropriate special training: but, as will be argued later, there may be difficulties in deciding what is appropriate. Lastly, the requirement of easy testing would exclude at least those propositions that can be only indirectly verified; that is, by inference and argument from perceptions.

These suggested requirements, indeed, are more rigorous than those that are accepted by the sciences and it does not seem that any psychologist would wish to do what the scientists find unnecessary. Stevens [66], for example, would apparently be quite content to accept as empirical propositions those which can be tested by an expert, in the laboratory, and which can be approximately verified by the accumulation of instances, so far as that may be necessary. However, it is possible to go much further in this direction also, away from rigorous conditions. Ayer accepts indirect verification [2, p. 14] on the ground that direct reference to perception is too harsh a criterion for the propositions of the natural sciences, and he also accepts weak or merely probable verification [2, p. 37] on the ground that requiring conclusive verification would exclude all kinds of inductive general law. But he goes beyond these common scientific tolerances. Historical propositions are to be admitted as empirical because they are capable of weak verification [2, p. 37]; i.e. they may be improbable or highly probable, but not certain. Further, a proposition is empirical if it is verifiable in principle but not necessarily in practice. Thus [2, p. 36], a proposition about the

D   37

geography of the back of the moon is admitted because a rocket could be made to take observers there; and historical propositions are admitted under this head too [2, pp. 18, 19], though it is not clear whether going back into the past is also to be regarded as a mere technological difficulty. An empirical (or verifiable) proposition, then, is one which could be tested by experience but it is not necessary that anybody should be actually capable of testing it now.

But this is a logical definition of the whole class of empirical propositions, which distinguishes it from the class of logical propositions but which does not throw any light on practical differences within the class. The question for psychology, in relation to its range of evidence from subjective and inexact but highly relevant to objective, exact and irrelevant, is what kinds of empirical proposition will be admitted. One may decide to admit all empirical propositions, or only those that meet the requirements of the sciences, or not even all of these. The easiest way of approaching this question is to set down the rather loose requirements that seem to be applied by most psychologists, though they may be too loose for the more scientific, and then to consider their consequences in practice. An empirical proposition in psychology, then, is one the operations for testing which can be specified and can be carried out by a trained psychologist under some actual conditions, although the test may be difficult, expensive and long. This merely reflects the fact that psychological investigations are made outside the laboratory as well as in it. Further, an empirical proposition is one which, when tested, can be at least weakly verified: that is, shown to have a specified probability which is below unity. Psychology obviously does accept very weak verification. In rare cases there is a sharp separation between the means of two distributions or a high association, however it is measured, between two variables; and in these cases the proposition, while it is not conclusively verified, is highly probable. In the usual case of 'just significant' differences or associations the probability that the proposition is true is low enough, whatever the psychologist's convention with regard to chance may be.

Besides this, the point is easily missed that in such a case only the rather vague proposition that there is *some* connection or *some* difference between the variables can be even weakly verified. Take the proposition that might be put by a student of psychology with sociological inclinations: that workers' occupations are 'determined by' their fathers' occupations. In a carefully assembled sample of 100 workers 50 are clerks and 50 artisans, and 32 of the clerks' fathers were clerks but only 18 of the artisans' fathers were clerks. Computing chi-square for the usual null hypothesis, the student gets a value of 7·84, with P less than 0·01. This he accepts as a weak, though conventionally quite respectable, verification of the proposition. But what his finding means is only that the moderate association observed is unlikely to be a fluke of sampling from a population in which there is really no association: and this is not at all the same as determination. It may be thought that this means only that the student should state his proposition more carefully. So he should: but there is more to it than that. A great many propositions in psychology are only weakly verified in the statistical sense; that is, far from tending towards conclusive verification, their probability is merely at the conventional level of significance. Now these are necessarily what might be called attenuated propositions: they signify that there is some association, for example, but not much. But they are the basis for the psychologist's verification, by inductive argument, of propositions of a higher order. He goes on to explain the association found or to discuss the relations among several associated 'determinants' of a variable and in doing so he states, though he may not explicitly test, further empirical propositions: for example, that filial succession in work is due to such and such patterns of family or social relations. These further propositions are obviously much easier to verify if they are based on clear and sharp findings instead of on the attenuated finding that something not very marked is going on, which is the usual case.

A similar difficulty is found when the psychologist wishes to transfer particular findings to similar but not identical cases. For example, he knows that there is a sex difference in performance on a particular test of clerical aptitude and he may wish to use this test on a different population (in another country, brighter, older, etc.) or to use a similar test on the same population. If he has to use the test for practical purposes before experimenting with it, then he must infer whether the difference found would hold in the changed circumstances. Not being shy of inductive generalization, he may make the inference quite happily, and perhaps even without noticing that he is including with the one verified proposition a number of unverified propositions, such as that the sex difference is not affected by intelligence or age. Such generalization is inescapable because many of the established findings of psychology are highly specific propositions: but a proposition which is generalized from a specific finding is obviously much more weakly verified, if it can be said to be verified at all, than is the original proposition. This will be true whether the original proposition is highly probable or merely 'significant', though the latter is clearly the worse basis for generalization.

It would appear, then, that propositions of any complexity or generality in psychology may be capable of only the weakest verification in so far as they depend on other propositions that are weakly verified and that are too attenuated and too specific to afford a basis for generalization. This amounts only to saying that behaviour is so complex and variable that testing hypotheses, if it requires no elaborate or esoteric methods, is bound to be a long and tedious task. This is obviously true with such a simple question as what determines entry to an occupation. As soon as one goes beyond the attenuated hypothesis that a single specified factor has something to do with it, to attempt an inclusive hypothesis that will take all the relevant factors into account, one strikes trouble. The relevant factors will include occupational level, age, sex, educational record, culture, economic conditions, parents' and sibs' occupations, family relations generally, the entrant's personality (a complex of factors by itself), special agencies (such as vocational guidance) and probably various others. This question could well be a life work for several large teams even though it is easy to investigate. It is to some extent open to deliberate experimentation, as the investigators could try the effect of different occupational counselling schemes in selected schools, using other schools as control groups. Where intervention is not possible, the selection of comparative evidence is always easy, for leaving school to take up work is something that everyone does, whatever his personality, family relations, education and so on.

It hardly needs remarking that the psychologist's operations are not always so easy to carry out. In some fields, notably in the study of frustration, deprivation, aggression and other kinds of unpleasantness, the manipulation of the situation is hardly possible. There are limits to what even the most masochistic disciple of science will tolerate and limits to what even the most devoted experimenter can reconcile with his superego or with the rules of his society, in his treatment of persons who are in his power (e.g. infants or patients). In these fields and in some others the psychologist must rely on what comes his way, so that his evidence may be rare and is likely to be fragmentary, making the assembly of comparative cases difficult. Besides this, there are large-scale events that cannot be manipulated and which may happen so rarely, or may extend over so long a period, that the psychologist may never be able to study their effects. The effects of war or economic depression on the choice of an occupation would be, one hopes, among the things the psychologist may be unable to study directly. Predictions, or empirical propositions about the future, referring to the whole course of a person's life (e.g. a statement of the conditions under which a schizoid character would deteriorate) may be incapable of test till the end of his life, if they can be tested then.

THE SIMPLE PROPOSITION HAS NO SPECIAL STATUS

However, if the simpler propositions of psychology are too attenuated and specific to afford much ground for generalization and if the more general propositions are too complex and unmanageable to be capable of easy verification, all of them are empirical propositions. The distinction between the propositions of objective measurement and those of psychology at large is not at all between empirical and non-empirical (or nonsensical) propositions, but merely between those that may be easy to test and those that certainly are not. For practical reasons, some propositions are hard to verify: not because they are obscure or doubtfully empirical, but merely because the operations required to test them (which can be exactly specified) may take years or generations of work by many psychologists instead of a few months' work by one experimenter in the laboratory. Meantime, a complex proposition is likely to be only weakly probable but when the work has been done there is no reason why its probability of being true or false should not be as high as that of a simple proposition. Presumably, then, all empirical propositions are equally admissible. Even the proposition that men will be twelve feet high at the end of history would be admitted, on Ayer's argument; for it will be testable at the end of history. That may be going too far, but the line must be drawn on practical grounds. Apart from definitions, there cannot be any propositions in psychology that are not empirical, except for those that are obvious nonsense because the operations for testing them cannot be specified: e.g. that the soul is spherical, translucent and elastic is not an empirical proposition. But if the meaningless is excluded, one must be careful not to exclude with it the proposition which is hard to analyse and understand. That an intense narcissistic need for personal approval is typical of the schizoid character may be hard to verify not only because of the complexity of the work involved but also because specifying the operations is rendered difficult by the terms of the proposition. 'Narcissistic need', 'schizoid character' and even 'personal approval' do not have self-evident meanings. None the less, it is suggested that such propositions, as well as the more obscure propositions of the psychoanalysts, must be accepted as empirical in so far as their terms can be analysed.

One could go further and observe that, as analysis means analogical reference to one's own real or imaginary experience, there is no ground for excluding even the most obscure propositions, such as those that might be derived from the poets. Ogden and Richards, indeed, distinguish sharply [53, p. 125] between symbolic words and 'symbolically blank but emotively active' words, and assert that the poetic use of the latter [53, p. 148] is 'totally distinct from the scientific use' of language. Their conclusion [53, p. 237] that there is a simple antithesis between science and art is much the same as that of Ayer [2, p. 44], that poetry is emotive, not factual. For the psychologist, this distinction is doubtful. Even so simple a statement as Dunbar's comment on the rich, 'And when their bags are full, their selves are bare', points to (or communicates) an experience more complex than a mere emotion. The same is true of Donne's conventional metaphors, 'My heart is by dejection, clay, And by selfe-murder, red'; and Blake's visionary declaration, 'In every cry of every man . . . The mind-forced manacles I hear', is not obviously unimaginable. If such propositions are thought to point only to the emotional experience of the poet, then this experience must be remarkably complex. It is, indeed, likelier that these propositions point to a highly condensed and abstract experience which is compounded of many elements, both emotional and intellectual. Maybe they are hard to understand because the poet's experience is harder to reinstate, or to enact in imagination, than is the experience which simple propositions point to. None the less, the poet's highly condensed propositions are ordinary empirical propositions; not, as Britton [6, p. 262] allows, poetic truths of a special kind, but empirical statements which are special only in that they say in a few words what might otherwise require several volumes. The distinction between factual (or empirical) and emotive propositions depends on a distinction between thought and emotion which is only logically valid; for there is no experience which cannot, and probably no complex and continued experience which does not, include both ideas and feelings. The psychologist, in fact, could perfectly well investigate the three poetic propositions quoted as hypotheses about human nature; and, if these, then any propositions of a more conventional kind, however obscure, complex and condensed they may be.

The only ground, indeed, for excluding such propositions from the actual field of psychology would be that they are so difficult to verify that the effort required is uneconomical. But considerations of practical economy would rule out the propositions of objective measurement even more firmly. Though these cannot claim a superior status on account of their uniquely empirical nature, they may be relatively easy to verify. But, on the argument of Chapter 3, they give no ground for building up more complex propositions. However much one knows about second signalling systems or factorial test abilities, one cannot infer from these to the determinants of entry to an occupation. Propositions in the field of common experience can be tested only in that field.

The choice for psychology, then, is between working with easily verified but largely trivial or irrelevant propositions and working with complex propositions in the field of common experience, which are fully as empirical as any but much harder to verify. Ever since the unfortunate discovery that language is richer and more complex than mathematics it has been fashionable in some circles to affect a kind of schizophrenic myopia and to draw a sharp line between those few not very human experiences that can be easily tested and reported and the rich but presumably terrifying variety of ordinary life. It is not apparent that this fashion need tempt the psychologist. Science itself is by no means so simple, transparent and unadventurous as the fashion would suggest and, in any case, the psychologist's profession allies him not so much with the scientist as with the ordinary person in the world. This person does not find much difficulty in testing the propositions which guide the conduct of his affairs. He is prepared to assert, for example, that the sun rises in the east without doing a series of experiments on it. He may be willing to meet the psychologist on some more special propositions and to say, for example, that family relations and the labour market must have something to do with entry to an occupation, while size of hat and annual rainfall are irrelevant. In making such assertions, he is drawing on his own experience of entering an occupation and of others doing the same: experience which the psychologist has too and which he can quite legitimately use. It may not be sufficient for a final test of the proposition but it is bound to give some degree of verification, for no proposition about ordinary human behaviour can be simply conceived in a void.

So much for the way the experimenter handles his propositions and his evidence or experience. There remains the question of relations between experimenters. If a proposition is empirical, the operations necessary to test it must be capable of a specification which can be unambiguously communicated to everyone who has the appropriate training. Now what communication does is to point to the experience of both parties and it is unambiguous if the person addressed can find in his experience, real or imaginary, a close analogue to the experience of the speaker or writer. If he cannot do this immediately, he may be able to try out the specified operation, so far as he understands the specification, until he does clearly understand it on the basis of his experience. Common professional training is therefore the necessary basis of understanding but it may not be sufficient, for in any field understanding may depend on specialized experience which must be developed by practice on the common ground of training. This development is trivial if the special experience required is perceptual, e.g. experience in handling apparatus. Where development depends on conceptual experience, it may not be so easy. Presumably it would take some time, and a little effort, before a physicist specializing in the thermodynamics of gases and one specializing in cosmic rays could understand each other's special propositions exactly; and the same would hold for a junior and a senior worker, though the difficulty here might be one-sided.

Now in psychology the experience which may have to be developed may be perceptual, which here too is a trivial case, and must be to some extent conceptual, which can probably be developed as easily as in other fields. But the psychologist's basic experience is personal; concepts may be derived from the analysis of direct knowledge of persons, including oneself but they cannot stand alone. Judgement, not abstraction, is the chief act of knowing, as Gilson observes [26, p. 297]. When a proposition points to experience of persons that the psychologist does not have, he can make up the deficiency either by going and getting experience, which may be tedious, or by constructing imaginary experience out of similar events that he knows, which is not very satisfactory. Or he can write off the difficulty as not falling within the scope of scientific method, which is concerned only with easily communicable propositions. This may be what Stevens [66, p. 27] intends when he proposes to accept only propositions: 'based on operations which are public and repeatable'. On the argument of Chapter 2, one person's knowing another, if it is an operation, is neither public nor repeatable in quite the same sense as is the person's knowing a percept or an idea. At all events, any proposal to restrict the acceptance of propositions as empirical is just as arbitrary when the ground of restriction is the difficulty of communication between experimenters as when it is the difficulty of any experimenter's verifying the proposition. In the former case as in the latter, difficulty of verification can rule out a proposition only on the psychologist's practical decision that he personally would rather not try.

The consequence is obvious. Persons who do not have the highly specialized experience which is necessary for testing some propositions may accept these on authority or may reserve their opinions indefinitely, but they cannot reject them, as they are not competent to do so. This is the force of the psychoanalysts' claim that their propositions can be adequately assessed only from the inside, by persons who have been psychoanalysed. There is nothing remarkable in this claim, which is implied throughout psychology, though it is never noticed, let alone stated, in the fields which depend more on perceptual and conceptual experience, as these are easily had. The general claim, indeed, is not remarkable; for the verification of any proposition is possible only for trained and qualified persons. Anyone who looks at an ammeter may be able to describe a naïve visual percept but the interpreted fact that the instrument is reading twenty milliamps can be reported only by someone who knows how ammeters work and what they are for; that is, by someone who has learnt certain special and quite elaborate conventions. Verification is in principle always a public process, as Ayer [2, p. 132] asserts with reference to the most general propositions about the nature of other persons: but the verification of any special proposition is possible only to a special public.

For most purposes there may be an obvious and universally accepted division between the majority who agree that they cannot test the proposition and the minority of specialists who agree that they have tested it and that it is sound, or not sound. But the advance of knowledge can hardly depend on agreement or on a majority vote among the specialists, for there may be disagreement even on who is a specialist. Where there is doubt on the experience that would be necessary to test a proposition, the only way to resolve the doubt is to keep on trying to test the proposition. The question of verifiability then passes from the present debate of logic into the continuing argument of history. If there is no finality in this, as Collingwood asserts [14, p. 180], then there can be no uniquely certain formal identification, either of the special public that is competent to test a proposition or of the special conditions under which a conclusive test would be possible. Even the most obscure and specialized proposition, therefore, cannot be ruled out as meaningless, let alone rejected as unsound, merely because one cannot say for sure by whom and under what conditions it could be tested.

The point of the psychoanalysts' assertion, of course, is that it is especially their direct acquaintance with patients in analysis, their judgements, which can hardly be assessed by anyone who has not taken special measures to have similar experience. Their concepts are much easier to assess as similar conceptual experience is within the reach of any psychologist: but, unless he has the primary, direct, experience also he cannot really test the propositions of psychoanalysis even though he may be able to undertake the logical analysis of its concepts. The objective verification of psychoanalytic propositions is primarily a task for the psychoanalyst. However, the difficulty need not be exaggerated. As psychology depends on common experience, the most special experience that is required in a particular field may not be so far out of the reach of anyone. With psychoanalysis, for example, anyone can check for himself, without a very profound self-examination, that the primitive irrational remains very effective in operating the defence mechanisms of his sober adult life; and so in less specialized fields.

The conclusion is none the less inevitable that not all psychological propositions, even though they are undoubtedly empirical, can be tested by everyone who is formally qualified as a psychologist. This again merely signifies that verification may be somewhat more difficult than it is in the sciences; which is not remarkable, as the person is somewhat more complex than the animal, machine or circuit.

The restriction also signifies that by no means everybody can be trained for any kind of psychological work, as Ichheiser [29, p. 42] insists. A wide, if vicarious, experience of life, good insight into one's own limitations and skill in personal relations are at least as necessary in the more personal fields of work as the formal qualifications with which alone professional training can be concerned.

THE PERSON IN THE WORLD

IF psychology returns to an open dependence on common experience, instead of an exclusive use of supposedly special evidence backed up by implicit reference to common experience, it thereby openly accepts the task of extending, clarifying and in places correcting that common experience. One then has to ask what this is. To say that it is the experience that everyone has of what persons universally and necessarily do is easy, but misleading. Nobody's experience is universal, and this definition would invite the equation of the behaviour of a particular period or society or locality or even individual with behaviour in general: an equation which is rarely implied in psychology now. A more popular line in psychology, however, is to imply that there is no behaviour in general: there are only these particular behaviours. Where generality or particularity is in dispute, the question may be settled by reference to the facts. Thus one may decide that aggressive behaviour, although it is learnt, is universal, while ostentation of one's material possessions is also learnt but is not universal. When the psychologist wishes to go beyond the description of how persons do behave to the consideration of how they came to be that way, and especially to the inference of how else they might have come to behave, he has to answer questions of this sort. Some particular answers may be easy to find but the general question, within what limits is behaviour learnt, is not easily answered. Psychology has naturally been more concerned with the differential study of particular facts and of the relation of these facts to particular environments than with relating its results to the general framework of human behaviour. It is this relation which needs examining and a suitable starting point is the general consideration of the person in his environment.

The most general characteristics of behaviour, or those modes of activity in which everyone necessarily engages, are easily specified. Everyone incorporates parts of his environment, expands himself or enhances his ego: and everyone also refuses incorporation, contracts himself and withdraws or retreats from his environment. Whatever scheme of propensities, action tendencies, traits or personality variables may be used, it is always possible to divide the whole order of variables into these distinct kinds, outgoing and retreating. This abstract generalization is therefore not meant to be a definition of new variables in yet another scheme; it is meant only to point to those general features of common experience which lie behind the particulars of psychology and which have to be clarified by analysis.

The first statement, then, may be taken further towards specificity. Expansion or outgoing behaviour may be co-operative, as when the person goes to meet another, to engage in common activity, and so on; or aggressive, as when the person acquires something at the expense of another. Expansion is usually either co-operative or aggressive, or both in the one train of action if the person is undecided what to do or if he is engaged with several others. Expansion can also be neither co-operative nor aggressive but merely solitary, as when the person enhances his ego in fantasy or, by himself, acquires knowledge or achieves mastery over an object. Most solitary activity, however, is merely a subsidiary phase in a train of social action, so that sustained solitary expansion is a rare limiting case. Withdrawal, on the other hand, is usually solitary for its purpose is to remove the person from what is perceived as a threat. It may be incidentally aggressive, when it has the effect of depriving someone of something he wants, whether or not the deprivation is intended. It may also be indirectly co-operative if the person, by his act, assists others to withdraw.

It follows that the general statement could as well be put the other way round. If expansion and withdrawal are taken as the most general abstraction from human behaviour, then one has to add that expansion is either co-operative or aggressive and rarely solitary, while withdrawal is solitary and only incidentally co-operative or aggressive. But it would be just as reasonable to take co-operation and aggression as the most general abstraction and then to add that the person may undertake either when he is expanding or, in rare circumstances, when he is retreating. Either general statement, in fact, can be reduced to a simpler form: the person necessarily seeks community with the persons and things and ideas around him, and also fights them, and also flees from them. Not only must he seek community, fight and flee at different times in the course of his life, he may do so in complex succession within the one train of action or even with regard to the one object and finally, in a sense, with regard to himself as an object.

This summary description of the person's engagement with the

48

world he lives in derives from common experience rather than from psychology in the special sense. It is, in fact, too abstract and general to be of use in psychology, for psychology is naturally concerned more with particular tasks, roles or achievements than with expansion generally and especially more concerned with particular defence mechanisms than with aggression or withdrawal generally. But if one takes the general for granted and studies the particular without any reference back to a more abstract ground, one may arrive at a rather unbalanced view of the general, whether stated or only implied. A more balanced view would require an examination of the relation between engagement generally and the particular engagements studied by psychology: and the best point with which to begin this examination is the development of the person's expansive behaviour.

EXPANSION AND THE DEVELOPMENT OF THE SELF

It is a commonplace that the infant's only expansive behaviour is the literal incorporation of things, which soon leads into symbolic incorporation as social behaviour develops. As Parsons and Shils put it [54, p. 17], viscerogenic needs develop into social-relational needs. Beyond this early and elementary stage, mastery over things, though not, of course, their direct incorporation, remains an important instrumental expansion. The adult's mastery over a wide range of things is important to him as a necessary means of sustaining other activities but is not of central importance in itself. If those play activities which are an accepted and necessary part of everyone's behaviour are centrally important, the person is likely to be regarded as an overgrown child.

Somewhat the same is true of the incorporation of ideas or symbolic knowledge. While this begins relatively late and goes on more or less incidentally or deliberately all one's life, it is for most persons always an instrumental activity. This is obvious with the basic knowledge acquired in the earlier school years, but is true also of the most elaborate knowledge acquired during professional training, for example. In the usual case, the person uses this to earn a living. He may indeed pursue further knowledge for the sheer pleasure of knowing and may even make a living out of this: but even in this case, where knowing may have little direct return into living, living comes before knowing in its importance to the person unless he is one of those who are better described as intellects than as persons.

The elaborate and general but usually not very clear knowledge that the person has of the society he lives in is instrumental in a rather different way. This knowledge may be regarded as what MacIver [41, p. 307] calls a 'value system' or what Sherif [61, p. 201] calls 'standardized concepts' of society: or it may be taken more broadly, as including social stereotypes, attitudes and social ideology. Whichever way it is taken, it is the person's engagement with the whole of his society: and it is important to notice that this engagement is symbolic and indirect, not personal and direct. That the person can have direct relations with only a few others is so obvious that it is not worth stating. On the other hand, now that social psychology is making good the great deficiencies of the psychology of the isolated person, one may as well take care not to go to the other extreme by default. Doubtless the social scientists, the politician, the public administrator, the trade union leader and so on do use their knowledge of society in their work. Doubtless other persons do so directly in some circumstances; in war, for example, or in an industrial dispute or on occasions of high political tension, the person may refer his general conduct explicitly and deliberately to his social value system. For most persons under ordinary conditions, however, and for many under any conditions, it seems unlikely that general knowledge of society is more than the limiting ground of other more direct engagements. It can hardly be more than this in the usual case in which, even if it is called knowledge, it is an unordered collection of attitudes, stereotypes, isolated facts and half-formulated ideas rather than a clearly articulated conceptual system. What the person probably does with it in any ordinary case is to take it for granted and then to tend to perceive only what lies within its limits. Thus the employer who believes that workers are lazy and the worker who believes employers are slave-drivers are both somewhat unlikely to see each other as distinct persons; but the facts of their actual engagement with each other can easily supersede these beliefs as a guide to action. Of course, the symbolic engagement makes a difference even if it is superseded, for co-operation on a ground of stereotypical distrust is not the same as co-operation on a ground of confidence, even if the distrust is more or less dissociated. One could go further and say that the symbolic engagement makes more difference where the parties do not even know each other's social opinions; a common complication of industrial affairs. However, to allow that the person's symbolic engagement makes a difference in all circumstances and that it makes all the difference in some is not to allow that it makes all the difference all the time.

The incorporation of knowledge, then, and even more the mastering of things are to some extent prior to and for the most part remain subsidiary to, the person's main or centrally important engagement, with other persons. As a mode of expansive behaviour, this differs

50

little, if at all, in earliest infancy from the incorporation of things. As soon as persons are differentiated from the environment, and as soon as the self begins to be differentiated, it changes radically. Whatever elements of plain object-relations (or incorporation or dominance) there may be permanently in the person's engagement with others, this engagement cannot be altogether an object-relation, simply because others are not objects, they are co-ordinate with the person. The person may engage with others as objects to dominate or instruments to use (e.g. to learn from) or because he depends on them for some particular purpose (e.g. protection in a particular case). But fundamentally he depends on them, as they on him, simply because they are other than him. The person depends on others, in relation of freely given love, for his very existence as a person. It may not be in the best of taste to use the word love, which just now seems to belong largely to certain fields of applied zoology: but some word is necessary to point to that quality of the person's essentially human engagement with others which distinguishes it from his other engagements.

That there is such a quality appears in many fields of experience. It is found even in the abstract consideration of communication as the means of learning, of which Mead [45, p. 69] observes: 'We take the attitudes of the other persons into our conduct', in responding to them. That is, we identify ourselves with them in some sense and do not merely learn to manipulate them as we would a machine. But this does not mean identification with the other person in all points, or simple imitation: it means a community of interests in which the persons remain distinct. Jaspers, on the same topic of communication in general [31, pp. 436, 437], puts the latter point forcibly: 'Ich will, dass jeder andere sei, wie ich zu werden mich *bemühe*: in *seiner* Wahrheit er selbst zu sein. Existenziell ist die Forderung: Folge nicht mir nach, sondern folge die selbst! Selbstsein erweckt Selbstsein, aber zwingt sich ihm nicht auf.'[1] Dufrenne and Ricoeur, commenting on Jaspers, stress rather the active community of interest in engagement [18, p. 122]:

'Je ne puis m'éveiller à moi-même sans y être appellé par un autre, lorsque son amitié est assez désinteressée et assez généreuse pour qu'il renonce à exercer sur moi quelque autorité, voire quelque influence, et qu'il se contente de m'inviter à être moi-même. Ainsi je deviens moi-même par la mediation et par l'example de l'autre. Mais cet autre à son tour, il n'existe que par moi.'[2]

---

[1] 'I wish everyone else to be what I *strive* to become myself: to be himself in *his* truth. The demand is existential: do not follow me, but follow yourself! Self-being arouses self-being but does not force itself upon the other.'

[2] 'I cannot wake up to myself without being called to it by another person,

These general statements are far removed from the particularities of daily life, but they point to the personal reciprocity which is so large a feature of daily life that one takes it for granted. It is found, at the least, in the occasional politeness of passing contacts, more in the lasting relations of colleagues and friends and most in the mutual help, society and comfort of the family. In all of these relations, there is something more than the prudent calculation of giving, conditional on self-interest; and that something more is essential, not merely an addition. Whether one invents a technical name for it or whether one simply calls it love, the fact is evident in everyone's common experience.

To say that love is universal is not to deny that the person may hate, fight or flee from others, even from the very persons he loves. The fact remains that love is the fundamental human engagement and, as one mode of behaviour among others, it is universal. It may be thought that the work of the social anthropologists contradicts this, but the apparent contradiction results merely from an over-concentration on particulars. It is true that the person's particular engagements vary considerably among societies, and the particular modes of love therefore vary too. In many primitive societies, for example, love within the family takes a very different form from what it does in white society as the family is very differently organized; but an obvious manner of love is still found. There are some primitive societies, certainly, in which the expression of love is so rigorously controlled by inflexible customs and rites that it can hardly be expressed at all. It is not clear that these cases should carry much weight, as they are very few. A more important consideration is that they are all societies whose physical environment and resources are poor. This is especially true of the people of Dobu Island, whose culture depends uniquely on universal and elaborately institutionalized hostility: but even this culture has an outlet for friendliness. Benedict [5, p. 186] observes: 'The individual in Dobu who was thoroughly disoriented was the man who was naturally friendly and found activity an end in itself.' More important than the mere occurrence of one person who was maladjusted to the society of this island is the fact that he was tolerated: while he was regarded as an outsider, his friendly services were accepted and he was not imposed upon. At the least, then, if one abnormal person is friendly, his normally hostile associates accept his friendship without directly returning it.

---

when his friendship is disinterested and generous enough for him to give up exerting any authority, or even any influence, over me, and for him to be content with inviting me to be myself. Thus I become myself by the mediation and the example of the other person. But the other person in turn exists only through me.'

The anthropologists rightly emphasize the particular differences and indeed contradictions among societies, which are such that a normal expression of love in one might be regarded with horror and disgust in some others. But these, however marked they are, are differences on a common ground. In some societies love is the person's centrally important expansive engagement. In others, and, it would seem, especially under the pressure of physical deprivation, the person's symbolic engagement with his environment is centrally important. In these societies the rigid rules of normal behaviour allow the person's expansion only within the narrow limits set by the two threats of a barren territory and competition from others. Love is so dangerous that it is rigorously controlled: but it is not abolished. Under any known and perhaps under any imaginable conditions the person sometimes gives himself to others simply for the sake of doing so. Giving is not incorporation or mastery: it is a mode of expansion which, because it is uniquely human, cannot be described even by analogy but can only be experienced.

There remains to be considered another important mode of expansive behaviour, the person's engagement with himself. As the infant learns that he is separate from his environment, so in due course the older person learns that he is a distinct and organized person, not merely a separate body. Mead [45, p. 136] puts it thus: 'The body can be there and operate in a very intelligent fashion without there being a self involved in the experience. The self has the characteristic that it is an object to itself, and that characteristic distinguishes it from other objects and from the body.' As Mead also makes clear [45, pp. 137–140], the self can only be developed in social experience, as this development depends on reciprocal communication with others. The self so developed is not, of course, an entity or mental capacity: it is merely how the person perceives himself. This includes how he perceives himself in relation to all his other, or external, engagements, with objects as well as with persons and society: for, as Sherif [61, Ch. 12] observes, the distinction between personal and social relations is merely a conventional distinction of degree. The person therefore perceives himself generally as related to his society through its standards, which Sherif [61, p. 201] calls: 'norms or values, which are special cases of the (standardized) concepts of his group'. He also perceives himself as related to various reference groups, as described by Sherif [61, Ch. 5], through his acceptance of their particular norms or values; and as related to various individuals and to informal face to face groups. In all these relations he perceives himself, as he thinks he is (that is, as he is from his point of view): as he thinks others think he is, which, as Ichheiser [29, Ch. 5] notes, need not be the same as he thinks he is or the same as other persons actually think he is; and lastly, as he would like to be.

The phenomenal self, or ego, is therefore a complicated and perhaps precarious development according to the usual account given by psychology. Even so, it may be suggested that this account is too simple, in two ways. Firstly, it may exaggerate the articulation, coherence or inner consistency of the self. The development of the self has been described largely from the point of view of the person who is trained in exact symbolic behaviour and careful analysis, not to say from the point of view of the middle-class intellectual. Other selves, not to say many selves, may well be less complicated; for the self can easily accommodate vague perceptions and inarticulate ideas, as well as contradictory elements which cause no trouble (as they may in the complex self) because they are separate.

Secondly, the usual account may also exaggerate the dependence of the self or person on social conformity. Sherif's argument suggests that the stability of the self depends in the first place and chiefly on the acceptance of the values or norms of reference groups of a rather general kind, ranging from large face to face social groups to the whole of society. Smaller groups, such as the family, are hardly mentioned except as generalized institutions. This view, which tends to imply the primacy of the person's symbolic engagements over his social engagements, may be true but it is assumed rather than demonstrated with evidence. The person may see himself as a citizen or member of a class or colleague or club member first and as a husband, father or friend only second, or not at all, if he sees his family merely as 'the' family of his society. Or he may see his engagements in the reverse order of importance; and it is even possible that persons differ considerably in how they see their engagements. These are empirical questions of some importance, which are not to be settled by general assumptions or by the use of partial evidence. A related difficulty is the assumption that, whatever the person's reference groups are, his stability depends on his *acceptance* of their values. This is indeed the definition of reference groups, in which the person is ego-involved, as Sherif puts it [61, p. 249], by 'enthusiastic incorporation of and willing conformity to the values of his reference group'. While it is doubtless true that stability depends on some kind of group membership, it is by no means obvious that this kind is necessary, or usual, or even common. Here again there is ample scope for individual variation. Besides that, one might suppose that 'enthusiastic incorporation of values' would be a characteristic of the person's actual engagement with his intimates rather than of his wider social relations or of his symbolic engagements with this society and with parts of it. Of course, in a society in which conformity is highly

54

valued as a defence against anxiety the symbolic values might determine or even supersede the personal values. In more flexible societies, there is scope not only for more individual variation but also for individual initiative in making values. The person does not only incorporate values into himself, he also changes them. As Mead [45, p. 215] says: 'As a man adjusts himself to a certain environment he becomes a different individual; but in becoming a different individual he has affected the community in which he lives.'

TENSION, AGGRESSION AND WITHDRAWAL

In due course, then, as he becomes aware of himself, the person is engaged with himself. This is a symbolic engagement, but is expansive in so far as it is active and creative, an engagement which is effective in developing the self. The self, of course, includes all engagements; the person's actual engagements with things and especially with other persons, as well as his symbolic engagements with a wide range of ideas which includes ideas of things, of persons and of society as well as of himself. If all of these were expansive engagements and, where that applies, co-operative, there would be little more to be said about the person in the world. But the person's aggressions are as evident as are his co-operative actions and his retreats are as evident as his expansions. Both, indeed, are inevitable.

In the first place, everyone is bound to encounter the simple difficulties of living in a very full and rich world. There are tasks he may wish to undertake which are beyond his capacity in any circumstances; things or ideas, for example, that he cannot master or incorporate because he lacks the strength, skill or intelligence. There are activities he may wish to pursue which in their nature exclude other desirable activities or which can be pursued only through a first unpleasant phase; in either case, the person can expand if he is willing to pay the price. Further, there are many activities that the person cannot pursue for lack of time: the whole world may be open to him, but time rushes past while he explores or incorporates his little corner of it.

These recurrent minor frustrations may be so obvious that they are not noticed in psychology, or, indeed, in common experience: for they may not be experienced as frustrations. The person may usually observe the limits of his abilities, manage his choices and plan his time. If he persistently does not do these things, he is called maladjusted; and the psychologist may be able to clarify the general mislearning which underlies his superficial incompetence. But no one is so competent that he never tries the impossible, even if he does so only to test its impossibility. This he must do. He cannot know what is beyond his capacity, or what actions are mutually exclusive or what cannot be done in the time, without trying and seeing for himself. Even when he has done this, he may be inclined to try again in the hope of pushing back the limits. On occasion, then, any person will tend to incompatible actions. He will tend to pursue and also to withdraw from tasks that are beyond his capacity; to pursue simultaneously tasks that exclude each other; and to pursue more than he can handle in the time. If this tendency to incompatible action is to be named, a simple name for it is tension. One can then say that some degree of recurrent tension within the person is inevitable because of the minor complications of the world he lives in.

These minor complications may be found chiefly, though not necessarily only, in the person's object-relations. There are more serious complications in his relations with other persons. He may have to compete with others for the limited supply of things that everyone wants, or to render them services he dislikes performing as a condition of his being supplied. The difficulties arising from material shortages, of weapons, tools, seed, water, food and so on, are obvious enough in primitive societies, many of which have systems designed solely to meet the permanent threat of serious deprivation. Similar difficulties are found in civilized societies in times of disaster or economic depression and more pervasively, if less obviously, at other times. Competition in industrial societies seems to be none the less real for being elaborately indirect and none the less keen for having as its object consumer goods that, at the extreme, the person may not even have time to use. More important than this kind of general conflict of interests, however, is the whole range of actual and daily minor conflicts in which the person engages in the home, school and place of work. These add to an impressive total in the most smoothly run life, and all are likely to produce tension in the person. Where two persons are engaged in incompatible or opposed actions, there is tension between them, and also in each if both are aware of the situation. If A hates B and seeks to destroy him, B is not tense unless he is aware of A's intentions, which he is likely to be. Further, there is ample scope for anyone to misinterpret or overinterpret a situation which is not really threatening or an action which is not intended as a threat; and that this kind of mildly pathological mis-perception is universal can easily be checked in common experience. In any case, the person will be tense because he will see the situation as requiring incompatible actions; for both defending his interests and giving them up are incompatible with his pursuit of the peaceful enjoyment of things.

The give and take of daily life, then, is another general source of tension. It may be thought that it can hardly be more important as a source than are the minor complexities of an over-rich environment, for the normal person can surely meet both kinds of difficulty equally well. In a prosperous society, this would doubtless be true if there were no conflicts between persons except over their object-interests: but this cannot be expected. The person's chief engagement is with others and the more this is a genuine personal engagement and not merely instrumental, the more is it liable to complications. There are circumstantial complications enough. For some purposes, the person may have to associate with others who reject or even attack him as a person. If this is still not so serious, as it would seldom be a permanent situation, it is none the less a much more direct threat to the self than are the minor irritations or conflicts of other relations. In any case, it leads immediately to what is by far the most important difficulty, the inherent contradiction between the person's major engagements.

The person's main engagement with others is love, the spontaneous giving of himself for the sake of giving and for nothing beyond that. Love, in this sense, may be as unknown to psychology as it is to the tradesmen who have appropriated the word, but it is to be hoped that this brief description points to an irreducible fact of common experience. Now loving persons is by no means easy. In a society which is busy getting things done, personal relations tend to be crowded out, so that the person, if he is at all aware of the difficulty, will find an incompatibility in time between his engagements which is no longer trivial but quite serious. Further, personal relations tend to become instrumental: the other person is used as a means to the mastery of the impersonal world. If there is a clash here because the person is not content with merely instrumental relations, the tension will be more serious. There may be no clash between actual engagements, and this may be even more serious. If the person is quite content to treat others as part of the object-world, as things to be mastered, then his main engagement is simply abolished, for direction of any sort, even if it is only the prudent calculation of the return expected for love, is completely incompatible with love. Prudent self-interest and negotiated agreement are no more love than is open dominance. The abnormal person, who is incapable of love, will be quite content with less than human relations with others. The normal person, if he does exclude from his life its most human relation, cannot exclude from himself the desire for it: and between this permanently frustrated desire or inarticulate and abortive project and his actual engagements there will be irresolvable tension.

At the least, then, some kind of clash among the person's expansive engagements is almost certain. For on the one hand the person depends for his very existence as a person on the mastery of his world, on taking it in, on enlarging and inflating his ego; and on the other hand he depends fully as much on selfless giving, which is in its nature incompatible with any direct and deliberate enlargement of the self. This fundamental ambivalence of the person will cause no trouble if he has enough inner strength to accept defeats, irritations, rejections and threats without anxiety. In any other case (that is, in most cases) it will cause trouble enough, whether its ground of action is directly in the field of personal relations (the ambivalence of love and hate) or whether it is displaced into the field of object-relations.

It may be concluded that, in handling his expansive engagements, the person will experience the tension of incompatible actions or projects somewhere in the range from trivial incompatibilities of time or place, through clashes of interest between persons to the inherent contradictions of his own nature. It is therefore only to be expected that the person's expansive engagements will be aggressive in some circumstances, if only as a means of warding off threats, and will also be abandoned or suspended from time to time, when the person judges it better to retreat. It would not be relevant to discuss in detail the wide range of adjustive techniques and defence mechanisms that are used to reduce tension. Krech and Crutchfield [36, Ch. 2] review three modes of adaptive and eight modes of maladaptive behaviour that are used in response to frustration. Cameron [7, Ch. 6] distinguishes twelve adjustive (or defensive) techniques and Fenichel [23, Ch. 9] lists one effective and eight pathogenic mechanisms of defence that operate at a relatively deep level. These summaries differ quite a bit in detail but all three make the same two general assertions about the person: that he manages tension either by attack or by withdrawal. When the person perceives an object as demanding action which is incompatible with his other interests (that is, perceives it as threatening), he may attack it directly: or he may persuade himself that it is not really threatening or that it is simply not there, or he may flee from it or give up and lapse into infantility, which last four are all modes of withdrawal.

Now, while these modes of behaviour can hardly be adequate for the reduction of tension, they are likely to be used by everyone. It may be true, as Snygg and Combs say [63, Ch. 8], that the adequate phenomenal self can accommodate all the perceptual differentiations that are presented by the environment; that is, can accept and integrate threats within a stable ego. But, if this is a definition of the adequate self, it must be taken with some reserve. There are few persons so rent internally with incompatible strivings that they collapse into sick incompetence or suicide and there may not be many more who can buy peace only at the price of attacking themselves. The normal person, however, may achieve only a precarious and approximate integration when he has to resolve severe tensions under pressure of time, with insufficient knowledge of the situation and even more insufficient knowledge of himself; and this he has to do often enough. Further, when he has done so, he may soon be exposed to another tension provoking situation and will have to do his work all over again. It would be remarkable if, under quite ordinary conditions of life, he made no use, or even no considerable use, of the quicker ways of resolving tension. All of these are inefficient and some are as effective in perpetuating tension indefinitely as they are in reducing its level momentarily. For the normal person, then, life is not unmanageably tense, but it is tense, in its nature and as an inescapable consequence of its being rich, varied, ongoing and creative; in a word, of its being life.

PSYCHOLOGY'S SIMPLIFICATION OF LIFE

This somewhat dramatic conclusion is far removed from the psychologist's quietly empirical analysis of abilities, interests, drives, prejudices, defence mechanisms and so on, but it is by no means irrelevant. These particular studies begin from, if they do not ignore, the universal features of life; for psychology cannot explain its primary facts. It can give no account of how they came to be as they are, it can only accept them as they are. Co-operative expansion, aggression and withdrawal (or love, hate and flight) are not the primary modes of human behaviour because of anything before them; they simply *are*. However, psychology is certainly competent to describe, analyse and clarify these modes of behaviour and doing this is, indeed, an important part of its task. The study of particular social or personal varieties of these general modes both derives from and supports the general description. The one can hardly be undertaken without the other. So far as psychology proposes to study the development of the self under particular social conditions, or the relations between expansion and withdrawal in particular cases, or the differences between modes of expansion and withdrawal or between ego-ideals that are approved in different societies, it must take account of those modes of behaviour that are not merely local but are universal. If it does not do so, it runs the risk of reducing the universal, either by the naïve error of supposing that the particular is universal or by the more sophisticated assumption that there are no universals beyond the particulars. It is not suggested that either of these views is explicitly maintained or even clearly implied by any school of psychology. However, the natural specialization of psychology does have the consequence that the practising psychologist, and even more the unwary student, may forget the general context of the particulars which are his special interest. The main tendencies thus to reduce the human drama to a spuriously simple form must therefore be considered.

The first of these is the empiricist reduction. In itself, the objective empirical study of the person shows only that he has such and such test abilities, aptitudes or motor skills; his engagements with the real world are simply ignored. This is quite legitimate for the special purposes of this kind of study, but may be rather limited for practical purposes. For these, what matters is not so much or at least not only how much intelligence, verbal ability or finger dexterity the person has, as measured by tests, but how far he can use the capacities in specified tasks. This will depend to some extent, perhaps to a large extent, on how he sees himself in relation to these tasks and in relation to other persons concerned with them. The ignoring of these ordinary engagements may be one reason for the relatively low efficiency of selection testing in many fields. A similar but more striking case is the empirical study of traits, attitudes, adjustment and personality variables generally. The person simply has these qualities; he is dominant or gregarious, prejudiced or conservative, socially well or poorly adjusted, and so on. The qualities measured are associated, but their dynamic relations are unknown, so that one has to assume that all operate in all situations. One cannot ask, for example, whether the person is dominant in frustrating situations, conservative because he is frustrated and poorly adjusted in situations that he cannot dominate. These particulars, and the relations between them, are left out when the person's ordinary engagements are left out and his world of many parts is reduced to a blurred and unordered background.

In its classical phase, psychoanalysis adumbrated two notable and complementary reductions. The first of these was the theory of instincts. In recent psychology generally, instincts are regarded in much the same way as in biology, as quite specific unlearnt modes of behaviour in which one response or a narrow range of similar responses is elicited by equally specific stimuli. Parsons and Shils, for example [54, p. 9], observe that the only innate needs are the viscerogenic needs, which are fairly specific in themselves though they are capable of a wide range of cultural modifications. Sherif [61, Ch. 2] limits his list of unlearnt biogenic needs or instincts to eight specific organic modes of behaviour (two of which are reflex) and one general mode, the avoidance of organic injury, the status of which he regards as doubtful. The psychoanalysts, by contrast, have at times regarded as instincts both specific organic functions and general modes of expansive and destructive behaviour; e.g. *eros* and *thanatos*. It is not clear that the latter (and certain other generalities) were ever seriously put forward as unlearnt, let alone specific, modes of behaviour and their present status is doubtful. Fenichel [23, p. 55], for example, cautiously describes instincts as primary drives, the physiological source of which is unknown; and he implies that some at least are unspecific and modifiable. However this may be, there is more here than a certain vagueness in the use of terms. It seems that psychoanalysis is not interested in the distinctions between universal but unlearnt and specific functions, universally learnt but general functions, and particularly learnt functions. Co-operation, aggression and withdrawal are doubtless learnt in the general sense (for the isolated person could hardly co-operate with, attack or flee from himself), and they are universally and necessarily learnt; but they are not instincts, not only because they are not innate but also because they are not specific. Confusion on this leaves the way open for the reduction of these primary modes of behaviour to simpler modes: and psychoanalysis has tended thus to reduce love to a biological function with a variety of expressions. This is a tendency, not an explicit formulation, and is at present less emphasized than it used to be, but is none the less misleading.

The argument begins with the thesis that anxiety is basically due to 'goal-inhibited sexuality', as Suttie [67, p. 213] calls it. This is doubtless true of some patients and may well be to some extent true of everyone. As a universal proposition, however, it leads to the conclusion that the patient (or any person) is an isolated animal whose bodily pleasures are his only important needs and whose distress can be relieved by adjusting his relations with a partner who is primarily a biological apparatus and is a person only incidentally, if at all. Of course, this exaggerates the mistaken emphasis of analytic theory, let alone of practice, which, as Suttie [67, Ch. 14] observes, is more human than theory. The fact remains that analytic theory apparently has no place for derived but autonomous social needs. Besides this, analytic theory seems not to have much place for primary and universal social needs; as Suttie [67, p. 216] puts it: 'The possibility of anxiety and aggression referring to associative and expressive needs and *their* frustrations is beginning to be recognized but with manifest reluctance.' If this is only a mistake of emphasis, it is none the less grave. It implies that the person's primary engagement with others is not love in its own right but is merely lust with a variable and complicated overlay of precariously derived politenesses. This view may seem natural in the somewhat depressing clinical

61

atmosphere, but common experience suggests that, if it is a limiting case towards which the person's fundamental ambivalence may push him, it is none the less not the usual case.

It must be noted, however, that the analyst's mistaken emphasis does not preclude a broader view of love. One must insist that genital primacy is *a* prerequisite of love (in marriage) and not, as Fenichel [23, p. 84] has it, 'the prerequisite'; and the distinction is as important as it is apparently slight. But Fenichel, in the same passage, has a fair idea of the spontaneity in giving of love in one context. In its more general reference, as mentioned above, this is a complex and obscurely expressible experience that is hardly within the range of easily tested propositions and that certainly cannot be stated in a form suitable for ordinary experimental test. It is not asserted, of course, that such an experience is universal in civilized, let alone in primitive, societies. It is asserted that this experience occurs, and is irreducible by analysis. One need not go as far as Scheler [59, pp. 191–193], who practically asserts that love is a mysterious something over and above the traits or qualities that are loved (cf. [59, p. 192]: 'Da bleibt immer ein "undegründbares" Plus').[1] It is sufficient to say that love cannot be reduced by phenomenal analysis to self-interest, however elaborated this may be. If this is so, then the nature and conditions of this complex experience are proper and very important empirical questions. If it is the weakness of the psychoanalysts that they take too simple a view of the conditions of love, at least they do not ignore it. This is more than can be said for the general texts on personality, most of which seem to take a rather abstract and attenuated view of the person's central engagement with others. Thus McClelland [40, p. 274] refers to love as a: 'central ideological complex', which may be an appropriate statement for the case he is considering but is hardly adequate as a general statement. Cattell [9, p. 339] apparently thinks that love is compounded of: 'the satisfaction of the ergs of mating, gregariousness, protectiveness, fear (seeking for security), and self-assertion (pride in the possession of another person), as approved by society'. If that is love as he finds it, very well; but even Scheler's analysis, inconclusive as it is, suggests that the phenomenon may not be quite so simply self-interested.

Reductive tendencies in social psychology can now be considered. The first of these is the tendency to see the person as an object which is pushed around in a field of force. This view is rather suggested by LaPiere and Farnsworth [37, p. 382]:

'Should he (the person), furthermore, by force of social circumstances be one of those few who are expected to provide some measure

---

[1] 'There is always something left over, the ground of which cannot be known.'

of individual leadership for others, success will depend on his happening to lead them in the direction in which they happen to be going. With some striking exceptions, the individual counts for little in the social scheme of things.'

This passage implies a rather curious view of the leader at a level of some responsibility. He apparently wakes up to himself when he happens to notice or is told that he is expected to lead, and he then hopefully tries to find the head of the column that is going to push him along. Leadership of this more than doubtful quality certainly occurs but is not the usual case. More effective leadership is rather taken for granted by Mead [45, p. 216], who observes that both leadership and genius are socially conditioned but are none the less unique and original. Sherif [61, p. 453], writing of a particular kind of leadership, accepts the fact of its effectiveness but is puzzled by it: 'We are not in a position yet to handle the puzzling case of the unique individuality with which the creative artist stands out from the rank of his contemporaries.' Personal maladjustment, he thinks, is a factor but cannot see why this sometimes leads to success but more often to failure. The crude view of leadership then appears to be that it is an accidental and rather unnecessary role that may be thrust on the person; and the sophisticated view, that it is a real, effective and important role, the derivation of which is obscure. Either view implies that it is usual and natural for the person to do what his circumstances tell him to do, including perhaps leading if that is what he is told to do; and that if he does do anything that is not obviously given in his circumstances, and especially if he does it successfully, this is surprising and perhaps inexplicable.

If this is the case with leadership at a high level, there will presumably be no more scope for the incidental leadership or initiative of daily affairs. At this level too it seems to be implied that the person passively conforms to what is expected of him. Sherif [61, p. 201] says that the person's 'reactions to social stimuli—his likes and dislikes, his aspirations and loyalties—are regulated by norms or values, which are special cases of the concepts of his group'. Parsons and Shils [54, pp. 17, 18] speak of the generalization of social-relational needs in response to what the loving adult wants, to the stage where 'what the adult wants for the child, the child comes to want for itself'. One need not overinterpret these passages, the emphasis of which is correct enough from one point of view; but they do not leave much room for individuality even in ordinary personal relations. Now persons are evidently singular (no phenomenal self is identical with another), so it would seem that in spite of this they see both personal and general social situations in a

63

uniform way; or, if their perceptions are not uniform, they suppress the diversity in favour of uniform action. Perhaps this is so. At all events, it is strongly suggested by Mounier's description [47, p. 351] of conformism: 'Apathiques devant l'action, conformistes dans les comportements sociaux, nous ne cherchons plus qu'à devenir invisibles à force de banalité, à replier toute avance de nous-mêmes qui nous exposérait à une affirmation dangereuse ou à un renouvellement de notre vie.'[1] But this suggests that conformism may be a special defence mechanism, and the suggestion is reinforced by Mounier's discussion [47, pp. 410–417] of the use of substitute behaviour, such as making gestures, promises and elaborate plans, instead of acting. Clearly there are circumstances where merely going through the motions of conforming will save the person trouble, so one may suppose that some actual conforming behaviour is due to the same motive.

Of course, this makes no difference to psychology's description of conforming behaviour: if it is found that nearly all persons conform to what is expected of them in nearly all situations, then that is a fact. But the interpretation of the fact is not so clear. If expansion is a universal and primary mode of behaviour, then taking the initiative or leading (which is an entirely co-operative expansion if the lead is accepted) is not inexplicable, it is to be expected. Conforming, on the other hand, may need interpretation. As a form of co-operation or love, it is obvious enough, but it has hardly been considered as a form of withdrawal; and this is a problem which social psychology can hardly afford to ignore, for there is no withdrawal without tension, even if the withdrawal reduces the level of tension. If the person really is an inert and uncreative reflection of his circumstances, the tension of this unnatural state is an important problem; and if the state has been wrongly described, the problem of correcting the description is equally important. It is even possible that the deeper analysis of conforming behaviour would lead on to the study of adjustment in the general sense, of the person's conformity with his own fundamental nature instead of merely in the particular sense of social conformity.

The other reductive tendency in social psychology may be disposed of more briefly. It appears in the emphasis on misunderstandings of various kinds as the causes of social tensions. For example, in discussing superstitions, delusions, prejudices and stereotypes as cognitive organizations, Krech and Crutchfield [36, p. 172] observe that

---

[1] 'Being apathetic in the face of action and conformists in social behaviour, we seek no more than to become invisible by means of banality, to withdraw every advance of ourselves which would expose us to a dangerous assertion or to a renewal of our life.'

they are important only because they 'differ so widely from the realities of the situation'. The implication is that these sources of tension between persons (and therefore of tension in the person) are the almost accidental product of poorly adjusted social structures, but the question of how the realities of the situation are assessed is not discussed. Sherif [61, Ch. 14] takes much the same line, though he notes some difficulties in deciding what is a prejudice. With regard to actual social relations in the factory, Maier [43, Ch. 1] rather implies that poor relations are due simply to misunderstandings that can be removed by training in seeing the other person's point of view and Jaques [30, Ch. 12], in his long account of a particular factory, implies much the same. Now all of these accounts are doubtless true as far as they go, and the authors themselves present no rash generalizations. None the less, if these particular psychologists have properly limited themselves to the field of tensions due to misunderstandings, and have done valuable pioneer work in this field, it does not seem that all social psychologists should so restrict themselves. Behind the tensions due to misunderstandings, there may be others that are due to a real clash of important interests. The clash may be obvious, as in the collision with Nazi Germany. Where it is not obvious, it may be mistaken for a mere clash of perceived interests. Ichheiser [29, p. 33 and *passim*] somewhat vehemently argues that group antipathies are often called prejudice in cases where they directly reflect the realities of the situation. Whether or not this is so, it does seem that social psychology might usefully investigate this possible confusion, in order to clarify its own ideas about social tensions. A more important point is that social tensions, whether general or local, are not the only sources of tension in the person. The person's own ambivalence before a world which is promising and demanding, yielding and repelling, at the same time, is probably the main source of tension; and this too belongs in social psychology, as it is in a sense the basis of society and doubtless has manifold consequences in social tensions.

Reductive tendencies in social psychology have been discussed at length, so it may be as well to restore the balance by concluding that this is the only specialization which is properly called psychology. Its paradoxical name is perhaps suited to its rather special concern with the psychology of generalized social processes (that is, of the person's conceptual engagements); and a consequence of this concern is that in social psychology as in the general texts on personality the person seems to have only rather detached relations with others. But the specialization of social psychology is due only to its late arrival on the scene and is already disappearing. Social psychology in the special sense is the natural though not very efficient complement of the psychology of the person in himself. In the general sense, social psychology supersedes or includes all specializations, for the person in himself is a person in a void. There is no person in a void; there is only the person at home, at school, in his place of work, among his friends, in his society and with himself. So long as social psychology can include the study of all these engagements (that is, of all the person's engagements) it will be simply psychology at large. The person may be generalized from his roles, in the sense that these are one drama; but he cannot be known as a person if the plot and script of the drama are thrown away.

THE PERSON IN HISTORY

TO discuss the person's engagement in the world without taking particular notice of his history would be very artificial. If his present engagement is a complex set of tensely related particular engagements, it is also an artificial abstraction from a continuous series of present engagements, in which each develops from the one before and into the one after. The account of development as a description of changes in particular engagements is correct as far as it goes, but it leaves aside the question of how changes happen, which involves the consideration of the general characteristics of the person's history. Obviously this too is in the background of the particular studies of psychology; if the person's present engagement gives the area of the background, his history gives its depth in time.

In the first place, the person's history is evidently not merely fortuitous. So far as it includes, as it must, what happens to him regardless of his actions, it is fortuitous from the point of view of psychology, but it also includes more or less of what he as an actor makes of events. Like an animal, he grows and declines physically. He becomes larger, stronger and capable of more precise actions and, after a long prime, weaker and less capable of precision. But it is not at all certain that intelligent learning, or adaptive behaviour, is subject to an absolute limit in the same way as physical strength and the basic motor capacities are. It is true that the person does not learn to solve more complicated crossword puzzles, of the kind that appear in intelligence tests, than he can solve by middle adolescence. However, it is uncertain how far this limit of development is innate and equally uncertain how far solving puzzles is related to solving the more complex problems of real life. It therefore by no means follows that the person is constitutionally unable to learn to solve problems that are more complex than those he can solve as a youth. Further, so far as the solution of the problems of ordinary life depends on accumulated experience, there is ample scope for

67

development, as these problems lie before the person all his life. At the least, then, he is bound to learn plenty in detail and can go on learning until he is overtaken by physical decay.

Now learning depends generally on changes in engagement. In any settled engagement, the person's picture of himself (that is, his phenomenal self) is more or less congruent with his picture of his situation, and especially with his picture of what others in the situation expect him to do or of what needs doing with things. In a new situation the person's learning by repeated and varied activity to bring his phenomenal self into line with the perceived requirements of the situation has the effect of developing habitual behaviour which, in a continuing situation, he perceives as adequate or satisfactory. This habitual behaviour is to be distinguished from the much less important occasional new responses that the person makes to transient situations, and may be so distinguished by calling it the person's style. Thus the person is energetic or slow in his work, abrupt or pleasant with his family, conservative or radical in his social opinions, cheerful or reserved with his friends; and so on.

In any fairly stable and continuing situation there is little tension in the person (though there is probably always some) if he has learnt adequately how to handle the situation; he tends little to incompatible actions or projects, that is, because his perception of the situation is congruent with his perception of himself. The simplest case of congruence is, of course, when the person enthusiastically identifies himself with the requirements of the situation, but it is not the only possible case. If the two sets of requirements diverge, there are various ways in which the person can handle this divergence, some more effective than others. One simple way is for the person to maintain a style of behaviour which suits him and to push past the situation. Thus a husband may spend most of his out of work time playing golf and much of his working time doing anything but the work he is paid to do. Ineffective though this obviously is, he may get by on the narrow margin of toleration of his family and colleagues. At the other extreme, the person may give up himself instead of the situation and may conform meticulously to what is expected of him, whether from a fear of particular consequences, or from a general fear of standing by himself. In this case the husband does as he is told at home and carefully behaves at work as he thinks his employer expects him to. In this case there is no tension between persons, while in the case where the person goes his own way regardless there may be plenty. None the less, this solution may be equally ineffective; for, even if the person only does things that he does not actually dislike doing, he necessarily relegates many of the things he wants to do to the permanent status of unrealized or even unformulated projects. His learning then proceeds on a background of suppressed tension instead of open war.

Between these two extreme cases there is the very common case where the person oscillates more or less rapidly between conforming and autonomy, whether as between roles within the day or week or in time generally or both. This also is obviously ineffective, as he probably has the worst of both ways. None the less, identification is not the only condition for effective learning. The person may be able to make an effective compromise between or synthesis of the styles appropriate to two divergent sets of requirements. A dreamily unpractical person, for example, may be able to learn how to be sufficiently alert, brisk and down to earth really to meet the requirements of his work or home, while he still goes on dreaming in the background behind his daily conduct of affairs. In the general case, as Parsons and Shils [84, p. 30] note, the person may creatively modify the behaviour which is socially expected in his role, in such a way that the modification is accepted. In this case he takes the lead and others conform, which is a quite ordinary event.

This gives the first condition of learning, which is simply what the person has already learnt; his handling, effective or ineffective, of his present engagements. The second condition is just as simple; it is change either in the situation or in the person. Change in the situation is bound to happen. At the least, it happens by mere lapse of time. The person grows and declines and so do his associates, and both he and they may move around enough for the association to change noticeably. Beyond this least kind of change, there is the inevitable but still actively personal change from one phase of the person's life to the next, when he practically must start work, for example, or retire, or when he may marry; when, at all events, he must decide what to undertake in the phase which is now open to him. Beyond this again is a sudden and particular change in his personal circumstances, as in the great love or great opportunity of his life, or in grief, sickness or bereavement. Finally, there are the changes of general disasters; if plague and famine are now confined to primitive societies, they seem to have been effectively replaced in civilization by unemployment and war.

Change in the person (that is, in the phenomenal self) is less obvious and is less to be expected because the whole aim of the person's learning is to hold the phenomenal self constant in changing circumstances. None the less, some change of this sort is to be expected independently of changes in the situation. For as the situation changes the person provisionally changes his style. The change may be slight or radical, but it is not final until in due course in the new situation the person can evaluate his change in style. Only then, which may be many years after the change in the situation, is there a final change in the phenomenal self, and this may be a single sudden change. The time comes when it is clear to the person that his style is successful and his phenomenal self is enlarged by the experience of success, perhaps gradually, perhaps suddenly. If it becomes clear to him that his style is unsuccessful, he may suddenly or gradually lower his aspirations, thereby shrinking the phenomenal self, or more probably he will gradually rationalize his failures and eventually come to see himself as a misunderstood or unlucky man. If his developing experience of the changed situation is not specially of either success or failure, it will still differ from his expectations in having clarity and definition. The phenomenal self of a man with even a few weeks' experience in a role, let alone months or years, is different from what it was when he provisionally entered the role. Krech and Crutchfield [36, p. 66] observe that the trend of behaviour often involves not merely a return to a stable equilibrium but the active integration of a more complex equilibrium. For important situational changes, at all events, this is obviously inevitable even if the integration takes years. No man, for example, can enter the major engagements of his adult years and remain a child; at all events, not without being quite inadequate to his engagements. The main process in active integration in this case is the revaluation of the past as the meaning of life emerges.

CHANGE

So much for the conditions of learning. It is now possible to consider how the person learns, or, to put it at length, to consider in what circumstances, given his already learnt styles, his changes in style in changed situations and any consequent changes in the phenomenal self, will or will not be effective. This general question may be approached by considering the main possibilities which a changed situation may offer the person, and how he may handle them. The simplest case is that of a change merely in the details of the situation. For example, when his firm moves the person moves his home to go with it or changes his employment to keep his home where it is. There may be numerous changes of detail, such as that the new home is more convenient in some ways and less in others, is in or near the country or in a country town instead of being right in the city, or that his new job has a slightly different status or rate of pay, is more interesting and so on. None of these will have much effect on the person. A change of style is not required, so there is no question of changes in the phenomenal self and equilibrium is easily

70

restored. The case is not quite so simple if the person has intimate friends in his neighbourhood or among his colleagues; but then he probably decides to stay with them, whichever move that requires. Even if he has to lose touch with one or the other set of friends, he can do this, not without sorrow, but without lasting changes of style. Learning in this kind of case is probably only incidental and is usually easy.

A less simple case is that in which the situation allows, invites or requires the person to take on more, wider or more responsible activities. This case may include aspects of all the changes that the person meets; taking on adult roles (such as his first job, marriage, fatherhood), advancing in these, as by promotion in his work, and even some disasters which offer scope for enlargement (as when war or the death of a member of his family increases his responsibilities). What the person does in this case will depend simply on how he sees the situation. If he sees it as one that he can cope with, whether or not doing so will be pleasant, he takes on his new responsibilities and begins working out or modifying his style. His learning proceeds efficiently by more or less deliberately guided trial and error, not without tension but without withdrawal, and in due course he reaches a more clearly articulated and deeper perception of himself. But the situation may appear to be a threat to the phenomenal self and in this case the person refuses engagement; he withdraws, maybe with concomitant aggressions by way of justifying his withdrawal. Obviously he learns nothing from experience of the new situation and although what he learns from his new experience of refusing engagement will depend rather on what it is that he has refused, it is bound to be inefficient. If he refuses to rise to an exceptional occasion, he may learn only a few distortions of the facts, both of the situation and of his own past; whereas if he refuses a normal but optional adult engagement the distortions will be more considerable, and he can hardly refuse the compulsory adult engagement of work without distortions so severe that he will be obliged to flee from society, whether into the asylum or the bush. In any case his perception of himself, once it has settled down after the upheaval of the tense period of refusal, will be distorted, defensive and rigid. The only exception to this would be where the person refuses an optional advancement, such as promotion in his work, because he thinks he could not cope and is quite happy not to try. However, this would be a very rare case as refusing a significant promotion would usually meet heavy social disapproval.

The third possibility is that the person sees the situation as one that he can and will cope with, but his role expectations, or the way he sees himself playing the part, are quite wrong in detail. They are out of line with the requirements of the role, whether these are in the

71

nature of the things in the situation, in the expectations of other persons concerned or in general social expectations. This may happen through ignorance, in entering an adult role; through rashness, in taking on a particular engagement in an adult role (marriage or work) without sufficiently detailed consideration; or through pathologically distorted perception, as when he dreams himself into a quite unsuitable job or marriage and then sits back and waits for a miracle to help him out. In the case of ignorance, the person's learning proceeds much as in the ordinary case of his assuming new responsibilities. Extreme ignorance, indeed, is a special instance of the ordinary case for everyone is bound to lack detailed knowledge of a task he has never done even if he can correctly imagine its general nature. Learning in the case of folly is also much the same as in the ordinary case though the process of trial and error is distinctly more tense and the person may indulge more often in occasional aggressions and withdrawals. Even so, he is likely to reach a similar deeper and well-articulated perception of himself; in fact, it is arguable that as he must learn by making mistakes, he will learn more by making big mistakes though one can hardly turn this possible result into a prescription for action. The case of pathological distortion, on the other hand, is similar to the ordinary case of the person's refusing engagement. All is well until his failure finds him out, as it must in time when the inadequacy of his behaviour can no longer be tolerated by the other persons concerned or (if there are no others) when his not having done the job he confidently proposed to himself to do becomes so obvious that even he must acknowledge it. At this stage, the learning of defensively distorted perceptions of the situation and of his own past begins, and it proceeds with a rush, for having been forcibly held off meantime, through to the new distorted and rigid phenomenal self.

To restore the balance of this somewhat abstract argument, it may be observed that the usual situation in real life is one that the person perceives as both promising and threatening, and in which he learns more or less efficiently according to the balance he manages to strike between success and failure and, underlying these, between expansion and aggression or withdrawal. It follows that the changes in the person's phenomenal self include both deepening and clarifying and also the strengthening of defences and the elaboration of distortions.

What the person does in a situation that invites or requires him to take on less, narrower or less responsible activities may be considered more briefly. This case may happen as the person reaches the later adult roles (when his children leave home and when he retires) or when he meets personal or general misfortunes (sickness, bereavement, demotion, unemployment, etc.). In any such case he will probably see the situation as threatening. He may then accept the threat and learn deliberately how to handle the new situation by working out substitute activities for those that he has to give up and remaking his perception of himself in the process. This is a difficult kind of learning and, depending on the situation, is perhaps unlikely. The person is likelier to approximate this process by trying various not very satisfactory substitute activities in a not very intelligently handled succession, and to develop some compensatory neurotic symptoms. This case differs only in degree from that of the person who moves rapidly into infantile substitute activities or neurotic illness or both; so that these inefficient kinds of learning are much the same as the person's learning in a situation offering wider responsibilities if he sees that as threatening. The same holds for learning in a contracting situation if the person misperceives it in detail. The longer he tries to behave as if the narrowing of his activities really made no difference, the harder he falls when he can deceive himself no longer.

PERSISTENCE

It may be concluded that learning, if it is at all effective, is an active, deliberately entered and intelligently varied process. Whether effective or not, it is active; it is the person's striving with his circumstances, not his merely receiving impressions. This is to say that learning is not a special process at all, it is simply the person's engagement in time, or his becoming. While learning is therefore in the present, it cannot be understood without reference to the person's past and future. The infinitesimal present is the imaginary moment in which the past becomes the future but the effective present of history is the period in which the person *changes* the past into the future. At the least, the extended psychological present must be taken into account, as both Lewin [39, p. 306 seq.] and Chein [11, section (ii)] allow; but describing this present may not be as easy as these authors apparently believe. In the present, the person refers the possibilities of the situation as he sees them to the expected future as he sees that. The future may not be seen in any detail and cannot be seen realistically where a big change is in question, for that the person can refer only to imaginary experience. But whether the person sees the future as a detailed plan or even a set of alternative plans or sees it only as a broad possibility, he sees in it what he wants, in some form, and he is bound to refer his present evaluation of the situation to this. Further, he may openly and deliberately refer to his past as he sees that, using it as a source of evidence for the evaluation of both the present situation and the expected future. Chein [11, section (iii)] at least allows that 'the present past' may be important in determining the person's action. However, this is still not enough. Whether or not the person actually refers to his past as he sees it, his perception of both present and future depends on his past. It is limited by the learning of the past, for he can only perceive the present and the future in the light of past experience, as summarized and generalized in the present. But this generalizing is not simply and uniformly derived from past experience, so that the psychologist always does well to use evidence about the person's past (if it is available) in order to understand his present. The person sees the present situation as an invitation or a threat, for example, because it seems to parallel his earliest relations with his parents or because it seems to be a particular case of a class of inviting or threatening situation as defined by the norms of his social reference group; or because of some combination of these factors. What he actually does will depend on which factor, or what combination, is operating. Where the person cannot himself refer to these factors in his perceived past, which would be the usual case, it is therefore the more important that the psychologist should be able to make this reference, though of course it will be to the person's past as he, the expert, sees it.

At all events, in making his future out of his past, the person does something which is presumably not an arbitrary but a logical development. None the less, it is a development, a change. If the person adapts to present changes, he changes his empirical rules of action and thence his style of habitual activities and therefore to some extent his perception of himself perhaps even to the extent of actively revaluing his past. If the person withdraws from changes in his circumstances instead of adapting to them, he none the less changes his perception of himself, and before that changes his style and empirical rules of action. In this case the changes are defensive, towards greater rigidity; even so, they may well include an active, if in this case mistaken, revaluation of the past. In either case, the person is obviously the same at all times but just as obviously he changes. As Allport [1, p. 102] put it: 'Every personality develops continually from the stage of infancy until death, and throughout this span it persists even though it changes.' Paradoxical as this seems, it is made somewhat easier to understand by being referred, not to the person, but to an abstractly conceived organization of the person, Allport's definition [1, p. 48] of which is well known. Parsons and Shils [54, p. 7] have a similar but much shorter definition of personality: 'the organized system of the orientation and motivation of action of one individual actor'. In order to see in what sense this dynamic organization of systems or organized system can

74

be said to persist while it changes, one must begin by considering the larger question of what one means by saying that the person persists while he changes.

If one refers this question firstly to the person's general development, the changes are obvious. The infant has no perception of himself, and from his first confused perception that he is separate from his environment to his organized and articulated perception of his adult self the person goes through several distinct and complicated stages. As he does so, he changes his style quite markedly and may do this again later, in passing through adult roles. None the less, the changes are within limits. They are changes of detailed interests or of particular relations with particular kinds of object, but not changes in kind in the person's major engagement. Thus the infant who behaves as if he feels threatened by the persons around him may attack them or withdraw from them or do both as well as loving them, and he goes on behaving in basically the same way in later life. He does not become secure, loving and spontaneous as a schoolboy or as an adolescent or as a family man or in his retirement. Neither does the infant who behaves as if his chief need was to be admired by the persons around him find satisfaction later in giving and loving. If psychoanalysis had not pioneered the understanding of such cases, the bare facts of those described as well as of the reverse cases would be sufficiently evident in common experience.

The argument may be taken a stage further by noting that the person most obviously persists and does not change in pathological cases. The aggressive schizoid fights his father in every job he manages to hold for a while, the hysteric remains a dependent little girl at work and then in the home, the compulsive scrupulously accumulates objects in his office and home workshop, the manic hopelessly flees the devil wherever he goes; and so on. In these cases there is little possibility of change. Apart from radical psychotherapy, the person changes for the better under symptom-reducing treatment or for the worse, perhaps regressing directly to infantile behaviour, under stress. But both of these are superficial changes which do not touch the person's style in his major engagements, as he is inextricably engaged with the past as perceived in the present. It may be noted also that in such cases personality is hard to define. From one point of view the person has an 'organized system'; it is intelligible as well as persistent. From another point of view it is permanently disorganized, for its major elements are in tension with each other.

It might be suggested, however, that if persistence is characteristic of the maladjusted person, who cannot change because he is unable to learn by getting to grips with his situation, change is characteristic of the normal person who can learn. The normal person certainly does learn the particular behaviour that is required by his various roles, whether it is required by the situation, expected by other persons or required as he sees it, or any combination of these. In this respect too it is notable that maladjusted persons learn little. They may learn to go through the required motions. A submissive person may learn to act the big bully at work, for example, if that is clearly expected of him; or a hysteroid may learn to be dependable and a remote and dreamy schizoid may learn to be practical. This kind of learning, however, is superficial and is usually easily seen through by the person's associates. Further, it is limited to the less intimate relations. It may be easy in casual social relations and possible in work, but it is much harder in the family. This supports the idea that persistence is a characteristic of the maladjusted; but the normal person's learning is subject to the same limits as is the maladjusted person's. The normal person is much more able to learn particular behaviour that is required in the situation so long as it is in character, and the maladjusted person cannot really learn this behaviour because it is not in character. Conversely, the normal person cannot learn behaviour which is not in character (i.e. is pathological) while the maladjusted person can learn the new details of pathological behaviour because it is in character. This only makes the obvious point that if a particular situation, such as a job, or if a whole society, require behaviour that the clinician would call hypomanic (for example), then the hypomanic can well learn the detailed behaviour required where the normal person cannot.

The conclusion, then, is that the person does change but not out of character. This is a strictly limited conclusion. It is referred to the person and not to personality, because of the general uncertainty of meaning of the latter word and especially because, if it does mean some kind of organization, it may not mean a kind which is universal. Secondly, then, the conclusion is referred to character, which means only character in the ordinary literary and dramatic sense. This use may more definitely point to an intelligible experience than would an attempt at quasi-scientific definition. Subject to these limitations, then, one can say that the person changes within the successively drawn limits of his character; changes in detail, that is, while persisting in general. The limits are those of the person's infantile social learning, narrowed by the learning of his school years, then by that of his adolescence, then by that of his adult years. Within any of these main phases, progressive limits are drawn more or less continuously and the major narrowing effect may take the whole phase to accomplish or much less. How or how much the person changes will depend on the change in the situation as well as on the limits of his character as already laid down. The changes made to meet major changes of phase are usually more far-reaching than those made to meet lesser changes of circumstance within a phase: and the changes of the earlier years are obviously more marked than those that happen later. On the other hand, there is no simple synchrony between phases as presented to the person and phases of development as experienced by him. It is therefore quite possible for a person to grow up, develop or change out of step with both his chronological age and his circumstances. A person who is presented with unusually large responsibilities at an early age may well develop an adult mentality long before he engages in the adult roles of work and marriage. Conversely, the person who has difficulty in learning often has a childish mentality even when he has been engaged in adult roles for some time. Short of the case that he never learns, he may make the definitive change to being an adult quite late in the appropriate phase.

What the limited conclusion means, then, is that the person persists while he changes in the sense that only he could have become whatever he is. He is now wiser, more alert, more stubborn, sillier, and so on, than he was ten years ago; but only he, having just that unique history both up to ten years ago and from then to now, could have become wiser and so on in just that way about just those particular things.

One must be clear, of course, that the person makes his history. He changes only within successive limits, of which he may have some understanding or none at all; but he always observes the limits, if only by crashing into them and withdrawing. And he changes, by empirical and active engagement with the world; by trying out his possibilities in the given situation and making his history, whether he is aware of it or not, in a continually renewed grappling with the world. 'The self', says Farrer [22, p. 229], 'is a continuous intellective and creative activity which proceeds by concentration into successive particular acts. It is the substantial connection provided by activity as such and studied under the name of will, which holds together the self as well as the act.' Of course, in acting the person is limited in his possibilities; as Jaspers puts it [31, p. 33]: 'Es ist eine meiner ursprünglichen Erfahrungen, dass ich nicht bloss da und nicht die Möglichkeit von allem bin, was ich sein Möchte, sondern dass ich mir auch *gegeben* bin als ein *Sosein*.'[1] But the activity is equally real [31, p. 47]: 'Ich konnte empirisch mein Sein als meine Anlage, mein Nun-einmal-Sosein Aufassen; für mich als eigentlich selbst ist mein

---

[1] 'It is one of my original experiences that I am not merely there, and do not have the possibility of anything I would like to be, but that I am *given* to myself too as a *particular being*.'

Charakter nicht ich; ich habe ihn und verhalte mich zu ihm.'[1] The same point is made more simply by Dufrenne and Ricoeur [18, p. 121]: 'Je suis ce que je me fais, mais je me fais ce que je suis . . . mon être véritable est en avant de moi, non en arrière; il n'est pas défini par ce que je suis, mais par ce que je décide et entreprends d'être.'[2] Not only is this duality of activity in engagement and accepting one's given limits present throughout life, it is precisely in the maintenance of active engagement that the person persists. Mounier [47, p. 593] observes: 'Le moi est identique comme on est constant ou comme on est fidèle, par un acte continu d'engagement.'[3] The person, one might say, changes because he must in order to persist, or persists because he changes.

This general statement, of course, does not rule out either the case that the person persists in withdrawal, not changing when he should, or the case that he changes in mere passive conformity, not persisting when he should. Both of these happen here and there and both may well happen to some extent in everyone's life; but it would be most misleading so to emphasize either that it appeared as the normal or natural case.

In the work of the psychoanalysts, a certain emphasis on the person's persistence is as natural a derivative of the clinical setting as it is a concomitant of the reduction of the person to the biological level. It need be no more misleading than the latter. Ricoeur [56, pp. 377–382], who allows that tracing behaviour back to its infantile origins is both therapeutically useful and true in a sense, points out that it is not the whole truth because the person's adult engagements are with adult objects, including persons, in their own right. These engagements, that is to say, are not simply repetitions of those of infancy however much they may be limited by the person's infantile learning: in any new situation, the person has some scope for intelligent self-management through active exploration, both of the situation and of himself.

The social psychologist's tendency to emphasize conformity has been sufficiently discussed in the previous chapter. It requires only the additional observation that conformity makes history either fortuitous or impossible. If history is made by a few leaders, whose active and continued engagement is itself inexplicable, then the persons who conform to the situations that the leaders present them

[1] 'I could conceive my being empirically as my disposition, my particular being now at the moment; for me as properly myself, my character is not me; I have it and I deal with it.'

[2] 'I am what I make myself, but I make myself what I am . . . my true being is before me, not behind; it is not defined by what I am, but by what I decide and undertake to be.'

[3] 'The self is identical in the same way as one is constant or faithful, by a continuous act of engagement.'

with have only a second-hand history. They do merely what somebody else expects them to do: which may be true of some persons, but is not at all how most persons perceive themselves in action. On the other hand, if everyone conforms to everyone else's expectations, then change and therefore history are impossible, except in so far as change may be introduced by physical processes.

The particular consequences of these possible mistakes in emphasis are perhaps not to be taken too seriously, as the mistakes are only possibilities. The consequences, in selecting evidence and methods of study and in drawing conclusions about the causes of behaviour, of the empiricist omission of history are more serious. For the empiricist, whether he studies animal or human learning in the laboratory or whether he collects test, trait and inventory measurements, the person has no history. He has, in the simplest case, a number of measured performances in the present which have no connection even with similar past performances; or, in the case studied by what is quaintly called developmental psychology, he has similar or different but still unconnected sets of these performances as measured at different times in his life. The one thing that the empiricist approach firmly omits is development. How the person's memory span, spatial ability, nurturance, neuroticism and so on actually develop in his continued engagement with the world is unknown. In consequence, their significance in the present situation cannot be assessed. There may be scope for the intelligent management of neuroticism or even of a poor memory span, if such trifles matter; but one cannot know in what cases there would be scope unless one knows how these qualities developed. Equally, there may be scope for variations in the use of test intelligence. If one knows only the test measurement, one may expect that two or more persons with the same measurement will behave differently in real situations requiring intelligence, but one cannot explain the differences. One may be able to do this if one knows also how they perceive the situations and especially if one knows how far, and under what conditions, they have learnt to behave intelligently.

THE PERSON AS CAUSE

IT has been implied throughout the account of the person's engagement generally, and especially of his history, that the person is a cause of his own behaviour. In a sense this may be obvious, but it requires discussion at length. There is a marked tendency to assimilate causality in human affairs to causality in physics, and the consequences of this tendency are evident both in the determination of methods of study and in the making of theories. The general consequences, in the false objectifying of the relation between the experimenter and the person, have been discussed already in other contexts and perhaps require no further notice. However, there are important particular consequences of the false objective approach which seem to derive directly from certain assumptions about causality; and these must therefore be discussed generally.

It is assumed, of course, that every event has a cause. The event X happened because of A, B and C, in the sense that if any one of these had not happened exactly when and as it did, X would not have happened. The series is not merely temporal, from antecedent to consequent, but causal, from initiating or determining to dependent. It may be presumed that no psychologist would object to this elementary general formulation; for, if he cannot demonstrate the necessity of the causal connection, he is obliged to assume it in the same way as anyone else who is not prepared to lapse into inactive scepticism. However, it must be allowed that tracing the causal sequence A, B, C, in human affairs is a difficult and complicated task. A simple and popular way of setting about this task is to assume an analogy with the physical causation of common experience. The tree fell because the boulder pushed it: the person responded to the stimulus of a change in the environment.

Now this is too simple, for the person thinks he chose how to respond or whether to respond, to use the naïve terms of common experience. At all events, he deliberated and did not respond immediately; and maybe he responded differently when the same stimulus, as it appeared, was repeated. It is the relation between stimulus and response that needs examining.

With reflex action, this is no problem. The actions of breathing or of the eyeblink, for example, are set off directly by the appropriate stimuli. Beyond reflexes, there are almost automatic actions, such as paying a tram fare, where the train of events is nearly as simple. Indeed, it is not obvious that the most complex behaviour really presents a problem. The person decides to emigrate, for example. It may not be easy to define the beginning of the train of events leading to this decision, but if an arbitrary beginning or precipitating stimulus is fixed, the remainder is easily set down. The person then thought about the idea, sought information, thought some more, discussed his half-formulated project, thought some more and finally decided. Besides acting and talking, the train of events includes a good deal of thinking; that is, of the person's complex responses to facts and concepts presented to him by the persons he consults and also to his own verbal and non-verbal concepts. In principle, the whole series can be laid out in exact sequence and in this sequence every term except the first and last is both a response to the one before it and a stimulus to the one after it. MacIver's third axiom [41, Ch. 1] that causation, in the sense of necessary history, is continuous is as true of complex series with simultaneous and overlapping events as it is of simple unit series.

The external view of causation is therefore too simple only in that it does not sufficiently allow for events within the person as part of the series. These events cannot be assumed to be one term only, the response, or one intervening term; they may be the greater part of the series and are so with complex projects in which most of the series is elaborate planning. Clearly these events must be studied just as much as externally observable events if causal series are to be traced. That they cannot be studied by external methods is no difficulty, following the argument of Chapter 3; but they must none the less be studied as determined systems. If every event has a cause, so has every event within the person. His deliberation causes later externally observable events, but is itself caused. The point is obvious and it may be that psychologists assume universal causation as a matter of course. None the less, the point is worth elaborating as there is some tendency in psychology to assume that only visible external agents can be causes.

Firstly, then, that the person will deliberate and how he will decide must be determined. The only alternative explanation is what has sometimes been called the free will of indifference but, as an explanation, this is unthinkable. The assertion that the person can choose as he likes may mean only that he chose as he did because he liked what he chose, which is merely a tautology. If the assertion means that he could just as well have chosen otherwise, that he only chanced to choose as he did, it is not logically meaningless for it could be verified by sufficient failures to discover the causes of his choice. But the proposition taken in this sense is heavily contradicted by common experience, in which one's own behaviour is nearly always known directly as caused. The case that the person has no idea what made him do that is too exceptional to stand as the normal case, even if mere ignorance were sufficient to dispose of a universal axiom. Besides this, it would be somewhat paradoxical if just human behaviour were uncaused. This would mean that the system that is apparently the most intelligent, orderly and comprehensible is actually the least, because it is fundamentally anarchic. This again is completely out of line with common experience, because even the person who decides that he will not decide but will toss for it or sit back and wait on events knows perfectly well that he is deciding not to decide and can give reasons for his decision.

Secondly, the immediate cause of the person's decision is obvious enough. It follows from the account of the person's history that deliberation is determined by the person's perception of his situation in relation to his desired future and to himself at the present. He acts as he sees his immediate highest good in the situation; and his seeing is determined by his past learning as well as by the situation. Working out this kind of causal series may be very difficult, whether for the observer or for the subject; but practical difficulty is no reason for assuming either that it is not causal or that it is not a relevant series.

The practical question, then, is how to isolate and analyse the causal series. While it may be true, as MacIver argues [41, Ch. 6], that it is not practical to trace a causal series backward indefinitely, it is equally true that the only series which is naturally isolable must include all significant events from the person's birth on. Birth is the only natural break in the series, before which another system was in operation; but presumably it would be necessary to distinguish significant from irrelevant events. An example will help. Why did the person get on the tram just then? Because he was going home, and he was going home because he works in the city but does not live there, and he works in the city because he is a lawyer, and he is a lawyer because he has passed the necessary examinations, and he passed these because he won a scholarship at the university. The causal series then divides; he won the scholarship because he left home at 8.50 in the morning to go to school on the day of a critically important lesson, and also because his early toilet training made him a hard and conscientious worker; and so back to birth, if desired.

Now none of these events can be ruled out as obviously irrelevant, in the sense that they belong to another causal series. In physical causation, the individual's whole history from the indefinite past leads forward in one indivisible nexus to the present. The personal series outlined differs from a physical series in having a definite starting point and differs even more in that it must include inner events. The person's intentions, projects, plans, aspirations, motives and perceptions are perhaps sufficiently implied in the account given but if this is incorrect it is by deficiency rather than by excess. None the less, it is obviously ridiculous. There are at least two large gaps in it. It may be true that he is a hard and conscientious worker because of his early toilet training, though hardly because of that alone. But other persons who are rigidly trained do not become hard and conscientious workers and some persons do grow up like this who are not rigidly trained. The link is suggestive but not sufficient. A more trivial, if still large, gap is the assertion that he works in the city because he is a lawyer. Plenty of persons in other occupations work in the city and plenty of lawyers work in the suburbs. This link too is insufficient. Besides the gaps, there is doubtfully relevant detail. It is unlikely that any one school lesson could be so important that if the person had missed it he would not have won a scholarship. Even if the possibility is accepted, one merely defers deciding where to draw the line, for one could then include the fact that on the critical morning he went to school by tram instead of walking, and so arrived fresh and lively.

Even a ridiculous series, of course, can be made respectable by statistical treatment. Thus if one knows that the person had an exacting toilet training, attended school regularly and is a lawyer, and if one knows also the appropriate associations, one can quote the odds on the person's being hard working and conscientious, getting a scholarship and working in the city. This is the method of the empiricists. It simply avoids the analysis of the causal series by substituting concomitant variations that can be used for prediction. The method therefore breaks down, for variations of the usual low degree of concomitance are of little use unless one can determine which determines which and, even if the degree of concomitance is exceptionally high, this has still to be inferred from a separate analysis.

CAUSAL ANALYSIS AND EMPIRICAL FREEDOM

This analysis proceeds in two stages. In the first, the causal series is isolated and its limits defined by the statement of an explicit comparison which is to be investigated instead of the comparison which is merely implied in all causal questions. This means only establishing an experimental hypothesis. MacIver [41, Ch. 5] argues that apt questions in causal analysis are questions about specific differences in comparable situations, including situations where actually doing an experiment is impossible. All that is necessary is to frame the question, or hypothesis, in such a way that both the situations and the differences are exactly described.

In the second stage, the data are analysed. One looks for all the necessary and sufficient conditions of the specific differences and not for a single cause, as Chein [11, section (i)] observes. These conditions include at least some of the factors in the situation, as the person sees them, and also some of his aspirations, ideas, evaluations, memories and so on. It is useless to try and omit these for uncertainty. MacIver's comment [41, p. 263]: 'The chain of physical causation does not need mind except for its discovery. The chain of social causation needs mind for its existence', shows that the analysis of intentional behaviour cannot be dispensed with. But, as was argued in Chapter 2, this analysis is quite straightforward in principle, if sometimes uncertain in practice. The psychologist, assuming that the universal aspects of the person's engagement in the world lie behind his particular behaviour, makes an analogical judgement of his intentions, referring for comparison to the behaviour of other persons and also, if only implicitly, to his own real or imaginary experience. MacIver [41, p. 391] describes this as: 'the task of projecting ourselves by sympathetic reconstruction into the situation as it is assessed by others'; and he makes it clear that this judgement of common experience and not the statistical analysis of evidence, is the critically important element in causal analysis.

How this perhaps disappointingly simple procedure works can be demonstrated with several cases, starting with the case discussed above. The full treatment of this would require that it be broken up into several parts, in each of which several specific questions might be asked. Thus one's final statements might include that the person is getting on the tram, just now, because he has finished his day's work by the conventional time for shutting his office: instead of the bus, because it came first or because the bus does not go his way: and so on. Or again, that he is a lawyer, instead of a doctor or a civil servant, because his interests, abilities and work expectations were so aligned that he made a considered choice of the law: or, he is a lawyer and not a process worker because he won various scholarships: and so on.

A more general case may be taken from work on the job preferences of children of school leaving age. A group of working-class boys who were asked to make paired comparisons of preferences through a deliberately mixed list of jobs ranked mechanics and electricians first, then some glamorous occupations (explorer, scientist), professional, clerical and some skilled manual jobs third and unskilled jobs bottom. They did this because the situation was nicely constructed to allow them to judge in terms of fantasy and of known and expected reality at the same time. Thus the glamorous jobs took a high place on pure fantasy, not being seen as real jobs at all; but they were overtaken by the skilled manual jobs with the highest prestige because these were the best real jobs that were conceivably open to the boys. Professional and clerical jobs ranked third, out of the usual order of prestige, because they were not really open to the boys, and the unskilled jobs went to the bottom because they were well enough known to be disliked, especially as most of the boys (at the time of the investigation) must have expected to enter this field.

This case shows that the sympathetic reconstruction of intentional behaviour may be quite complicated even when it derives from a neatly planned investigation. As one leaves the directly experimental field, the complications naturally increase. It may be possible to say, for example, that the person is always dour, reserved and harsh at home instead of genial, as at his work, because he sees his family as threatening him and his work as inviting his expansion: or because his work frustrates him and his home behaviour is a controlled release of aggression: and so on. Such inferences, however, require at the very least a close and detailed comparative study of the person in all his present engagements, and preferably also a study of his history, as well as similar studies of other persons. These extensions from the purely experimental approach are even more necessary if one wishes to know why the person is as he is now generally, let alone if one asks why a group of persons or a whole society is as it is. In the last case, of course, one leaves psychology for general history.

None the less, it may be concluded that causal analysis is always possible in principle where specific questions about comparable situations can be framed. Analysis of any case may be difficult enough in practice for, as MacIver [41, p. 368] observes: 'We should not be satisfied that we have reached the causal nexus unless we have adequate evidence of the psychological process.' The more general the case and the longer its duration, the greater will be the practical difficulty. But the only question which is outside the scope of the comparative method (in psychology, at least) is the question why all persons are as they are; for the hypothetical differences that this would require are beyond even imaginary experience.

If causal analysis is always possible except in this limiting case, it is only a matter of time and labour till the determination of human behaviour is completely understood; and the person's belief that he is free in a sense in which things and animals are not is merely a temporary and ignorant illusion. The important question here is that of the practical limits of causal analysis, but as this is closely related to the nature of the person's illusion of freedom, this latter may be considered first.

It is obvious that the person has open to him a wide range of possibilities of action in his various engagements. If one avoids the vulgar error of supposing that he has complete freedom of action (in the perhaps rather misleading sense of freedom from external constraint), there is no reason to fall into the opposite error of regarding him as the creature of circumstance. Important as it may be to note that many persons do live in very constrained circumstances, as Sherif [61, Ch. 4] emphasizes, it is equally important to note that in the most threatening situation there are at least two possibilities open to the person. Even in extremity he may decide (it might be misleading to say choose) to endure or to perish. While there may be only two possibilities open to any particular person in a particular situation, the range of possibilities is wide enough in most situations for persons generally. Animals have a much smaller range and things have no range: they are completely determined by the situation. The difference is important enough to be insisted on even if the person's inference that he is free is a mistake, or a poor choice of terms.

At all events, the person probably exaggerates his freedom from constraint in the general case as well as in his own case. As the possibilities of any situation are completely determined for any one person by the situation and his perception of it, the possibilities for persons in general must be limited to those that are due to their differences in perceiving the situation, or, behind these, their differences in general knowledge, knowledge of themselves, intellectual ability and so on. These differences do not range so widely that great differences in action are to be expected.

However, this is determination in general as the psychologist sees it from the point of view of a detached observer; it is not at all how the person engaged in action sees himself. He may have the illusion that he is free in both of the popular senses; undetermined and unconstrained by circumstance; or he may be well aware that he is limited in the possibilities open to him and know, in a general way, that his actions are determined. He does not and cannot know exactly how they are determined, for he is constrained as much by his own ignorance as by circumstance and his ignorance in a sense sets him free, for it is the inevitable ground of his action. This is put briefly by Jaspers [31, p. 191]: 'Ich aber muss wollen, weil ich *nicht* weiss. Nur meinem Wollen kann sich das dem Wissen unzugängliche Sein offenbaren. Nichtwissen ist der Ursprung des Wollenmüssens.'[1] The person has to experiment in self-determination in order to know his own determination or, to quote Jaspers again [31, p. 331]: 'Nun muss aber gehandelt werden *bevor* das rational objektivierende Verständnis an sein mögliches Ende kommen kann.'[2] The person has to act on provisional generalizations and shaky hypotheses, derived from an obscure knowledge of his past, a quite limited knowledge of his present situation and an even more limited knowledge of himself, and from an insecure estimate of the future. He may know that he is determined but he certainly does not know his determination.

Of course he revises his generalizations and hypotheses as he acts, for in action he learns more of his determination. The relation is described thus by Mounier [47, p. 355]: 'Nous ne connaissons pas la réalité en l'attendant sur place comme une chose due, ni la réalité du dehors ni notre propre réalité. Nous ne les recevons, l'une avec l'autre, que dans l'effort que nous faisons pour les métamorphoser.'[3] Even so, the person can never completely know his own determination. As was argued in Chapter 2, the practical difficulties of knowing one's own present (or phenomenal self), let alone one's past, are considerable. They may even be so considerable that one could infer an absolute limit from the suggestion made by Dufrenne and Ricoeur [18, p. 124]: ' . . . il apparâit que l'existence échappe à la compréhension. Mais par excès, si l'on peut dire, et non par défaut: l'existence est trop riche, et non point, comme par exemple la matière brute, trop pauvre pour être comprise.'[4] Now the practical difficulty of seeing through the sheer complexity of one's existence leads to a more serious limitation: that the person's understanding

---

[1] 'However, I must will because I do *not* know. Only my will can reveal to itself the being which is inaccessible to knowledge. Not knowing is the source of having to will.'

[2] 'Things must be done *before* the rational objectifying understanding can reach its possible conclusions.'

[3] 'We do not know reality by waiting for it on the spot like something due to us, neither external reality nor our own reality. We only get hold of them, the one with the other, in the effort which we make to change them.'

[4] ' . . . it seems that existence eludes understanding. But by excess, if one can say so, and not by deficiency: existence is too rich to be understood, not at all too poor like, for example, crude matter.'

of himself and of his determination is never final but can always be upset by new experience. At any time, the person is unlikely to have much understanding of his determination unless he understands his history as well as his present. But as he enters a new engagement, he may actively revalue both his immediate past and his remoter past; that is, he arrives at a new, if not necessarily at a more correct, understanding of his determination. He may thus progressively change his understanding of himself whether by clarifying it or distorting it or he may not actually change it at all. But it is always possible for him to do so, and to do so actively, for as long as he lives he is not a closed system about which the last word has been said but a person whose existence and potentialities are not known until they are realized in action. It follows that no one, however insightful he may be, can fully understand his determination till the end of his life: for any new experience may throw new light on any phase of his life. Experience, indeed, is bound to illuminate the person's understanding of himself so long as he strives for this, as Dufrenne and Ricoeur observe [18, p. 121]: '. . . si ma recherche est authentique elle me met en face d'un moi en quelque sorte absolu: le moi qu'à force de négations, et quelquefois dans l'angoisse, j'enfante au long de mes actes, c'est précisément celui que j'avais à être, qu'au fond j'étais sans le savoir encore'.[1]

If there is no finality in the person's knowing his own determination, whether this is of his whole life or of any part of it, a consequence of the first importance follows. Like animals and things, though to a lesser extent, he is both determined and constrained by circumstance; but, unlike them, he is empirically free, for unlike them he can seek his determination in action. This is the difference which is perhaps evident in common experience and which underlies the obstinate use of the word freedom for a condition which the person himself acknowledges is also determined. But empirical freedom is quite compatible with determination. As MacIver says [41, p. 240]: 'Freedom is a way of being determined that is different from the way of coercion.' Different, that is, because it obliges the person to experiment, to find his determination in action. 'Le cœur de la liberté', Dufrenne and Ricoeur observe [18, p. 143], 'n'est pas tant dans le parti que je prends que dans le fait que je prenne parti.'[2] Jaspers puts the same point more emphatically [31, p. 182]: 'Im Entschluss erfahre ich die Freiheit, in der ich nicht mehr nur über

[1] '. . . if my search is genuine it confronts me with a self which is in a way absolute: the self that, by means of denials and sometimes in agony, I give birth to throughout my actions, is precisely what I have to be, what at the bottom I was without knowing it yet.'
[2] 'The heart of freedom is not so much in the decision I make as in the fact that I make a decision.'

etwas, sondern über mich selbst entscheide, in der die Trennung nicht möglich ist von Wahl und Ich, sondern ich *selbst die Freiheit dieser Wahl bin.*'[1] Jaspers, of course, is speaking of choice in the sense of empirical decision and it is important to note that the person's freedom in this sense extends over all his fields of activity. Ricoeur [56, p. 450] makes this clear:

'Dire oui reste mon acte. Oui à mon caractère, dont je puis changer l'étroitesse en profondeur, acceptant de compenser par l'amitié son invincible partialité. Oui à l'inconscient, qui demeurel a possibilité indéfinie de motiver ma liberté. Oui à ma vie, que je n'ai point choisie, mais qui est la condition de tout choix possible.'[2]

The person, one might say, is obliged to suspend judgement and then to consent and to act, in order that he may come to judgement.

HISTORICAL ANALYSIS IS NEVER FINAL

Now if the person is limited in his understanding of his own determination because he is free to explore it, the experimenter is doubly limited. As a subject, he is limited in the same way as everyone else: he can understand his own general determination only in action and never fully. But his understanding as an experimenter of the person as a subject depends critically on his use of analogical judgements, on his referring the subject's behaviour to his experience of similar behaviour in other persons and ultimately to his own real or imaginary similar experience. These analogical judgements are as likely to mislead him with regard to the subject's general determination as they are in lesser matters. Of course he can try to get round this. If his understanding of his own general determination is critically limited, he can still try to improve his understanding of his particular determination in understanding the subject. Every psychologist who pauses to ask himself just why he reached such and such a conclusion or who compares his opinion of the subject now with his opinion a year ago, is trying to improve his understanding. But if understanding in general is developed only in close, active and

---

[1] 'In decision I experience freedom, in which I decide about myself and no longer only about something, in which the separation of the choice and myself is impossible, but I *myself am the freedom of this choice.*'

[2] 'To say "yes" remains my act. "Yes" to my character, the narrowness of which I can change into depth, accepting the compensation of its invincible bias by affection. "Yes" to the unconscious, which remains the indefinite possibility of motivating freedom. "Yes" to my life, which I did not choose at all, but which is the condition of any possible choice.'

continuous engagement, then the psychologist's particular understanding of the subject will also require this kind of engagement. The logical dilemma here is insoluble. If the psychologist's relation with the subject remains brief and impersonal (as it must in practice) and in a sense abstract (as it must in most cases, where he can see the subject only out of his natural context) then his understanding remains limited because he is not closely enough involved with the subject. If, on the other hand, he is on intimate terms with the subject his understanding is limited by his own emotional involvement, in the same way as is the subject's understanding of himself: for in this case the experimenter is a subject too as well as an observer.

It may be that under the best conditions, when the experimenter has continued and active but detached relations with the subject, and even under some poorer conditions, the experimenter knows the subject better than the subject knows himself. In some cases, obviously, the gain in clarity through professional detachment outweighs the loss of evidence through remoteness. This one would expect to be the case if the subject is heavily involved emotionally with himself; if, as is usual, he consults the psychologist because he is in some marked difficulty. In other cases, the experimenter may know the subject as well as the subject knows himself but is hardly likely to know him better; one would usually expect the subject's superior knowledge of himself at least to balance, if not to outweigh, his lesser detachment from himself as an object.

So the argument returns to the limits of causal analysis and the conclusion is that, in its nature, causal analysis is possible only within definite practical limits, whether it is made by the person himself or by a detached expert. Causal analysis in psychology is rather like the efforts of a man swimming in a heavy sea to imagine what the shore looks like from an aeroplane a mile up. Whether the swimmer is just an ordinary person or whether he has been specially trained in this kind of imagination may matter a lot for various special purposes, but for general purposes it makes little difference, as both men are in the swim together.

Now in the sciences the experimenter is detached from his material and has control of it, while in psychology the experimenter has to try and control his material although he is immersed in it. This difference has some interesting consequences. The generalizations of psychology are limited, compared to those of the sciences. They are limited in scope because of the size and the range in time of the phenomena to be studied; in clarity, because of the complexity of even small scale phenomena; and, where causal generalizations are attempted, these are further limited by the difficulties of causal analysis. However, if psychology is in a sense limited because it is so much smaller than its object, this only means that it is not a complete science now, not that it is not a science in its nature. But it would seem that psychology can never be complete because it is a history and not only in history. The sciences, of course, are also in history. In any science, new discoveries may lead to new interpretations even if they are discoveries about newly investigated aspects of relatively unchanging objects or processes. On the other hand, so far as the objects or processes that are studied do change, the science must change when it has available data that were previously not within its scope. Such changes would not necessarily invalidate the generalizations of an earlier stage and they are irrelevant to the status of the science, which has the task of explaining the observed present only, not the possible future. But with psychology the case is not quite so simple. The time scales of cosmic and vital changes are incomparably longer than is the historical scale of the scientist as a person; but the scale of history is, if anything, shorter than the psychologist's scale, for events flood past him while he tries to understand them. The changes in the object of psychology, the person engaged in the world, are so rapid that psychology is likely to be overtaken by the next situation or phase or development long before it has finished studying the present one. The psychologist can no more stop history while he analyses a section through it than he can stand outside history to make the section. He has to revalue the incompletely understood generalizations he has achieved, in active engagement with a changing object, in just the same way as the ordinary person revalues his non-professional generalizations.

One could say, indeed, that the psychologist has to do what the historian does in order to understand the past by re-enacting it, as Collingwood says [14, pp. 282–302]; and he makes it clear that this is the same process as is required for understanding oneself [14, p. 219]. The psychologist's difficulty is that he has to achieve an understanding of other persons (and of himself: the procedure is the same) under almost impossible conditions; not in the dead past but in the rapidly changing present. That there is no finality in historical analysis in the strict sense may not matter, but for the psychologist's analysis of contemporary history it may be serious. Because psychology is immersed in its object, the dependence of its causal analysis on the empirical freedom of engagement is as effective with successive generations of workers as it is with the single worker, and, in his field, with the ordinary person.

It must be allowed, of course, that the difficulties of causal analysis are in proportion to its scale. Laws of strictly present behaviour which are systematic and not historical, and indeed non-causal laws, may be properly studied and applied by psychology. The discussion of the general usefulness of these laws and of their relevance to the development of psychology must be deferred to Chapter 12 onwards. Certain practical consequences of the tendency in psychology to write off the person as the agent of his becoming remain to be discussed here.

CONFUSIONS IN PSYCHOLOGICAL PRACTICE

It is rather assumed that the experimenter knows much more of the person's determination than the person himself does. Even if the person is the agent of his becoming, he does not know how: causal analysis is possible only for the experimenter, who is in this respect privileged by his professional competence.

In general, this may be only a slight exaggeration, if it is an exaggeration at all. It is true in psychoanalysis, for example, the reason for which is that the patient cannot know his own determination until he has actively engaged with himself under the direction of the analyst. It may be fairly true in general social psychology, for the quite different reason that the person does not usually think, and may not have the knowledge required to think, about his place and functions in society; so that the experimenter is relatively privileged by his learning. The experimenter's privilege is most obvious in empiricist psychology, and for the same reason. The psychologist's test and instrument measures of the person's behaviour are data so specialized that the person cannot understand them or relate them at all to his ordinary experience, and, if he tries to do this, may complain that it is impossible. In this case, however, the experimenter does not use his data for a causal analysis of the person: he abandons causality before he begins work. This contrasts with the situation in the newer fields of applied social psychology, as developed by Jaques [30] and Maier [43] among others, and in the phenomenal approach, as described by Snygg and Combs [63]. In these, the experimenter so guides the role-playing or the interview that the person takes the initiative in exploring his determination.

The contrast is reflected in other fields of applied psychology, in which the empiricist engaged in vocational selection, for example, or in the external methods of psychotherapy, directs the person's actions as a non-communicating source of power; while in vocational counselling, client-centred therapy and psychoanalysis the emphasis is on the person's empirical self-determination. Of course the distinction between these two kinds of procedure is not so sharp as this simple description suggests, and in practice the two may be combined. It would be irrelevant, even if it were possible, to discuss the practical merits in various cases of the two procedures. What does need discussion, however, is the confusion in defining what the procedures are required to do, or the complete lack of any definition, that follows from confusion about the person's status as the agent of his becoming.

The most striking case of confusion about results is a convenient illustration. This is the empiricist assumption that the treatment of mental disorder (that is, of the psychoneuroses and functional psychoses, or simply of emotional disturbances or disorders of behaviour) is something that one does to the patient and the success of which one assesses by reference to his immediate symptoms. Thus Spence [64, p. 77] says of therapeutic treatment that: 'it requires a knowledge of what to do to the individual, what changes in his physical and social environment to arrange, in order to bring about the desired behaviour changes'. Eysenck [21, pp. 25–32] has shown that as many patients recover after being given medicine by a general practitioner or after a stay in hospital without special treatment or merely of their own accord as recover after psychotherapy: so that the question of what to do to the patient is open as far as efficiency is concerned. Hebb [27, Ch. 11] similarly observes that shock treatment and surgery have proved value whereas psychotherapy is only hypothetically (though probably) effective.

The general implication is that, on the grounds of efficiency and economy, the physical treatment of disorders of behaviour, or even no deliberate treatment, is to be preferred to elaborate psychological procedures. This view may be backed up by the idea that disorders of behaviour are themselves in a sense physical. Thus Hebb [27, p. 263] hopes: 'that a contributing organic cause will be found for all those cases that are now called purely functional', and he points to the work on the constitutional basis of schizophrenia in support of this hope. Eysenck [21, Ch. 5] demonstrates a constitutional basis for his factor of neuroticism as measured by tests.

This empiricist approach to mental disorder involves a dualistic confusion between behaviour and its neural basis. It follows from the argument of Chapter 3 that disorders of behaviour are undoubtedly physical in a sense. They are purely physical in that they *are*, and are not merely based on, disorders of cerebral systems or circuits, even though these disorders cannot now be imagined, let alone described. But disorders of behaviour are also purely mental, in that they are not due to foreign physical agents, such as poisons, bacteria or gross lesions. The systems or circuits are as they are because the cerebral input (whatever that is) from the sensory receptor areas and the association areas made them as they are by repetition. It follows that these disordered, or dissonant or conflicting, cerebral systems cannot be ordered or made consonant or harmonious by killing bacteria or removing poisons, but only by a means equivalent to their cause. In principle, this could be done by a direct physiological input that would exactly untrace the original traumatic input step by step. What this would be like one cannot even imagine, so that one has to fall back on the behavioural or psychological input of ordinary experience.

It then becomes clear that the duality of the experimenter's point of view, as between his relation with the person as a person and his relation with the person as a physiological object, by no means implies a duality of process or of treatment. From the point of view of psychology, the person has learnt his disorderly behaviour. He has learnt, for example, to fear all persons who appear to have paternal authority, to fear women or to fear the dark. As the experiences in which he learnt these modes of behaviour are now inaccessible to him, he can unlearn his behaviour only if he can integrate the repressed memories with the rest of his learning. This Ricoeur [56, p. 376], with reference to psychoanalysis, describes as: 'un triomphe de la conscience sur ses propres interdits par le détour d'une autre conscience déchiffreuse'.[1] The patient, Ricoeur says [56, p. 367], makes a memory, perhaps a partly fictitious memory, out of what was only a vague something disturbing him. At all events, he achieves an integration of the repressed experiences with his present experience and with his perceived past and he can do this only by reactivating the repressed experiences under the guidance of his interpreter and then working through them until he understands them. When he has done this he is cured, in the sense that he will never again fear the objects he used to fear, any more than he fears other unthreatening objects.

Doubtless it is hard to test whether or not the person is cured in this sense, but the point to note is that by any other treatment he cannot be cured in this sense. Rest, a change of circumstances, advice on self-management, reassurance and permission to retreat into medicine-taking may all be quite effective in reducing his symptoms. They may allay his fears sufficiently for him to be able to return to his work and his family and carry on without a major breakdown. Eysenck and Hebb do not claim that these methods do more than this, for this is their criterion of cure. Neither do they notice that this is quite different from the cure which they say is achieved no more efficiently by extended psychotherapy. The symptom-reducing methods do not touch the cause of the person's disorders of

---

[1] 'A triumph of consciousness over its own prohibitions by a turning through another consciousness that decodes.'

behaviour; indeed, they are not aimed at the cause, and they may be used in the belief that the cause is inaccessible. At all events, because they do not touch the cause they have nothing to do with relearning or integration and they cannot therefore be said to effect a cure in at all the same sense as to methods that depend on active relearning.

The case with treatment by physical or chemical assault is the same. This kind of treatment either reduces the disorderly cerebral systems to a harmless level by a gross assault or simply amputates them, though it must be observed that the psychological situation of submitting to assault probably has a separate effect in some cases. These methods are even more irrelevant to the cause of the disorders of behaviour, for they bear no resemblance to the hypothetical equivalent direct cerebral input and they are not even very reassuring to the patient. They are therefore equally incapable of a cure in the radical sense of relearning, however effective they may be in reducing symptoms. The correspondence, in all cases, between treatment and consequences may be demonstrated by analogy. If a person has not learnt to walk, the obvious treatment is to teach him to walk: and this and this only cures him of his disability. If, for whatever reason, this cannot be done, there are other possibilities. He could be exposed to a grave physical danger, in the hope that the shock would suddenly teach him to walk, and if it did he would certainly be cured. However, if learning to walk were so difficult that ordinary teaching was out of the question in such a case (that is, as difficult as unlearning phobias) the shock would doubtless not teach him, and so would not cure him, even if it did teach him, for example, to crawl much faster than his usual speed. Alternatively, he could be taught to manage without walking, by using a wheel chair: but this is not a cure at all.

The other irrelevance that is implied in the empiricist's indifference to learning as the cause of behaviour disorders follows from the demonstration that these are in some sense due to heredity, and it can be disposed of briefly. It is not claimed that either the actual disorder or the neural basis is directly and simply inherited in the same way as, for example, certain kinds of idiocy, albinism or haemophilia. Kallmann [34] cautiously observes of schizophrenia that some kind of predisposition clearly is inherited, but that there is ample possibility for avoiding the disorder in spite of this and for contracting the disorder without this. The point here is that the cause of schizophrenia, in the proper comparative sense of those conditions which distinguish schizophrenics from others, is the learning of the years of infancy together with a constitutional predisposition. To omit learning as a cause would make nonsense of both prevention and treatment. Psychotherapy may be less effective with a patient who is predisposed to the disorder, but as he learnt it he may still be able to unlearn it: and the training of the persons who are charged with the upbringing of the predisposed so that they will be able to avoid making their behaviour a reinforcing cause is obviously relevant. Of course, if the predisposed person must inevitably become schizophrenic there is nothing to do but to leave him until he is ready for assault; but it is not asserted that this is so. The person who is born an albino may be taken as an analogy here. Unless one assumes that he must inevitably contract severe sunburn, which is ridiculous, one would look after him by advising his parents to keep him out of the sun and advising him to wear a hat, avoid sunny climates and so on; that is, teaching him and his parents how to manage his constitutional predisposition to sunburn.

It may be concluded that because the person is the agent of his becoming or a cause of his behaviour, it may make a critical difference in the results of treatment whether the person is treated as a causal agent or whether he is treated merely as an object. That it must make a difference in the kind of result is clear. Whether the difference in kind in the results of psychotherapy is important, is not known because it has not been investigated; but equal gross efficiency is not a sufficient ground for deciding between methods. Doubtless there are very strong practical grounds for using the object type of treatment with some disorders, and there are similar grounds for preferring the non-communicating direction of the person to a joint causal analysis in, for example, educational and vocational selection as opposed to guidance. The choice between methods on practical and moral grounds is not in question, nor is it in question that this choice must include considerations of efficiency, economy and so on. It is argued, however, that this practical choice should not be confused by a false assumption of identity in the results. The consideration of efficiency must take into account the fact that the results, far from being of the same kind though differing in degree, are distinctly different in kind. It is a logical defect of the empiricist approach that it cannot take note of this difference in kind because it rejects causal analysis altogether.

THE NATURE OF PSYCHOLOGICAL ENQUIRY

THE argument now moves from the consideration of what psychology should investigate into the discussion of how it should do it, a question which one need hardly say is of great practical importance. The function of psychology is not to supersede common experience (which is impossible) but to expand, correct and clarify it. The psychologist, therefore, must investigate behaviour which is not accessible to common experience, behaviour which can be studied only by a specially trained person using special methods. Besides this, however, the psychologist must study behaviour that nobody else has the time or the means to study adequately. The chief limitation of common experience is not that it excludes some experience, whether the repressed or the merely disapproved; serious as this is, it is only a special case of a general difficulty. The person who is engaged in the conduct of his affairs in any field is obviously committed to studying his conduct and that of others only in so far as this study facilitates action. He is committed, that is, to getting results at the cost of some lack of understanding of how he gets them; and, if he must try and detach himself from events to the least extent which is necessary for him to control them, the pressure is always on him to detach himself no more than this, if so much. This is equally true of the psychologist in his professional field, where detachment from the world of events in which he plays a small part is strictly impossible. However, his professional work is the study of other people's actions. He can give his whole time to studying what they can study only hastily or momentarily, in the press of action, and that for the psychologist is a relative detachment. But, as events move on regardless and the psychologist too has limited time, his methods must be economical to use and fast as well as technically adequate. A psychology which used methods chosen for their precision regardless of their expense or the time required to use them would not only be of little practical use, it would also be incapable of relation to the greater part of common experience, as this would move rapidly away from psychology. To elucidate the laws of human behaviour requires one to study events while one is immersed in them, and this requires one to use methods that are fast and economical, as well as precise.

This prescription may imply that psychology is concerned primarily with ordinary behaviour in the real world, and it is certainly assumed that psychology's ultimate function is to assist in the understanding of this behaviour. However, it does not follow that psychological enquiry must be directed immediately and solely to such behaviour. It follows from the previous argument that enquiry must be directed in some sense to the person's behaviour as he is engaged in the world, and to that behaviour interpreted with regard to his intentions, not merely observed. It follows also that empirical propositions (or hypotheses) of any size and complexity may be accepted for investigation, not only restricted empirical propositions. But these further prescriptions leave the main questions of method untouched, as a great variety of methods is possible within the limits proposed. A psychological investigation may cover wide areas of ordinary behaviour, or one area only, or a small part of an area. It may be directed to the person's actual ordinary behaviour, or to his hypothetical behaviour, or to his behaviour in an abstract situation. It may depend on open and flexible or on sharply defined and invariable procedures and it may go through to a simple or to a highly sophisticated statistical analysis. Finally, the report on an enquiry may relate the results to possible differences among investigators, or it may ignore these.

In all these respects the method must be suited to the matter to be studied. But different methods give apparently very different results. One therefore has to consider how far various methods may be regarded as simple alternatives, or equivalent, or irreducibly different; in general, how far the results to be expected from different methods are interchangeable or transferable. This question is taken up in the next three chapters with regard to the more important features of methods generally. The following review is introductory to these chapters and also disposes of certain features of method that do not require extended discussion.

The most obvious feature of method may be considered first; that is, the mode of behaviour to be investigated. Five main areas of ordinary behaviour may be distinguished. These are the person's relations with his family (including parents as well as his own family), with his friends and with his colleagues; his work performance (the actual task, whether physical, conceptual or social, as distinct from social relations incidental to it); and his relation to his society (conceptual). This is a loose classification, which could well be either extended or simplified. It would be quite reasonable, for example, to subdivide the person's social relations further and to divide his relations with his society into those directed to his social class and those directed to the whole society. On the other hand, it would probably be as reasonable to class relations simply as directed to persons, ideas or things. Any of these classifications would serve to bring out two important points. The first is that the study of the person cannot be reduced to a study of his relations. If his relations in the areas listed are narrowly defined so as to include only his actual behaviour in these areas, some subsidiary behaviour (e.g. his journey to work, which does not clearly belong to any area) will be omitted and so will some important underlying behaviour. The account of his family relations, for example, will include what he does at home, but not his general opinion of his home, or his general ideas about the family. On the other hand, even if the difficulties of narrow definition are avoided by broadening the areas to include subsidiary activities and deepening them to include the intentional and conceptual ground of the person's behaviour, there is still an irreducible residue. The person has relations with himself, in that he does things not only by himself, in the sense of subsidiary or instrumental activities (such as chopping firewood or writing a book), but also for himself alone, in various play activities and especially in daydreaming, brooding and ruminating. Whether or not such activities can be regarded as a sixth area, this would not be an area in the same sense as the other five, for some element of self-directed activity is likely to be found in the person's behaviour in all these areas. He may play with the guillotine he operates, for example, at the same time as he turns out the job; or he may enact a private daydream at the same time as he confers with his boss.

Secondly, the classification of behaviour by areas is incomplete because it omits behaviour which occurs only in certain special constructed situations, in the psychologist's office or laboratory. This kind of behaviour is better considered in the discussion of substantial abstraction, below; it is mentioned here in order to point out that, if it is considered as a seventh area of enquiry, it too is not an area in the same sense as the first five. For the other distinctions between areas, the question of interchangeability can now be put, and can be briefly answered. It is, one hopes, a commonplace that findings are not interchangeable among the five ordinary areas. Actions and ideology may or may not coincide, so that social behaviour may or may not be related to (or due to) social beliefs.

Behaviour in the field of work may be uniform in a generalized sense (e.g. the worker is meticulous or erratic both in his various personal relations at work and in the handling of his machine) or it may be varied (e.g. the worker is servile to the foreman, stand-offish with his mates and careless at his task). There is no need to multiply examples, for it may perhaps be assumed that the generality or specificity of habits or styles is a question that can only be settled empirically. Much the same is true for the relation between self-directed activity and activity in the five ordinary areas. Whether the former includes all covert behaviour or (more reasonably) only certain, as it were autistic, kinds of this, its relation to externally engaged behaviour is by no means obvious. The person may enact his daydreams in public, in parallel with his private fantasies, or only in private, in antagonistic compensation to his public behaviour; and so on. This too is a question that can only be settled empirically.

The first conclusion, then, about the nature of psychological enquiry is that in principle it must include the detailed study of wide and complex areas of ordinary behaviour. The magnitude of the task so proposed is hardly reduced by considering what kinds of behaviour should be studied in these areas. Behaviour ranges from habitual (the person's routine in the daily to yearly cycle of his life phase) to occasional (things he has done, or that have happened to him, once only). Psychology has been mostly concerned with habitual, or at all events with recurrent, behaviour; and this is reasonable, because the inference of general causal laws must be based on such behaviour. However, the general laws of habitual behaviour are not the only laws with which psychology can properly be concerned. Exceptional events, which may be of some importance in the person's life unless that is singularly monotonous, are doubtless lawful and may therefore have to be studied as carefully as recurrent events; and this may enlarge the scope of psychological enquiry almost as much as the concentration on recurrent behaviour reduces it. Further, the study of both kinds of event may require attention to the person's history. Obviously there cannot be either recurrence or exception in the immediate present and no psychologist would object to including a few years of the perceived past in his field of study. But from there to studying the whole of one phase of a person's life or the whole of his life is a long step, and from studying the perceived past to studying the person's history as it goes on, is an even longer step. None the less, these steps may have to be taken. Whether or not the general laws of past and present are interchangeable (so that only one set need be known) and whether or not the laws of recurrent behaviour are interchangeable with those of exceptional behaviour, are questions that must be deferred to Chapter 11. It is sufficient to note here, as a second conclusion, that psychological enquiry may have to be further enlarged to include the person's history in some detail. And even that is not all. The wider the range of the evidence, the easier it is to infer causal (that is, intentional) laws; for causal analysis, even if it is supported as far as it can be by persons' statements of their intentions, depends, as Snygg and Combs [63, Ch. 3] remark, almost entirely on the comparative analysis of events. But this need not be confined to the comparative analysis of the behaviour of isolated persons, conducted by one psychologist. Besides studying groups of persons in their own right, psychology might well study each person from as many points of view as possible. Following Ichheiser's suggestion [29, Ch. 5], one would then include not only how A and B see themselves, but also how they see each other, and so on for as many persons as possible. Further, one would include the counterpart to how the psychologist sees them; that is, how they see him. Whether or not it does make a difference which investigator carried out a particular study is another question that can be deferred to Chapter 11. The possibility is there and, together with the possibility of including detailed cross-evidence, it would give a third enlargement of the scope of psychological enquiry.

ECONOMY, RELEVANCE AND KINDS OF HYPOTHESIS

So far, then, it appears that psychological enquiry can extend and anticipate the knowledge of common acquaintance only in so far as it tends towards the breadth, duration and multiplicity of common acquaintance. For extension and clarification, this might be an unfortunate necessity, but for anticipation it very nearly means that psychology is not in the race, a somewhat unpromising conclusion. The answer may be found in the consideration of the short cuts that have been elaborated by psychology.

The first of these may be called *instrumental definition*. Whatever method of investigation is used (e.g. interview or test) and in whatever area it is used, the particular questions or items may range serially in definition. The least defined is the question (it could hardly be a test item) which may be presented anywhere in order, in any form of words. This is followed by questions with fixed wording, and then by questions (or items) with fixed wording and a set of responses for the person to choose from. This range may be regarded merely as a matter of working convenience; it is quicker to pin the person down to the point. On the other hand, it

H   101

is possible that the evidence got by these methods is not interchangeable over the range. In anticipation of the detailed discussion of this in Chapter 10, it will be sufficient to give two examples of the kind of problem that is implicit here. A questionnaire with multiple choice answers may or may not give a reasonable representation of the answers that would be got in an open interview. Even with a test of intelligence or aptitude, one cannot be sure without investigation that the official right answers, as selected, give as good a representation of the ability being tested as would the range of freely produced answers.

In any case, even if the person's responses to the investigator are to a large extent defined by the instruments used, not much is gained towards making the investigation manageable. The second short cut, *substantial abstraction*, may therefore be used. In any area, the enquiry will not include every last detail of what the person did, but will concentrate on general or recurrent behaviour. This may mean only that the enquiry is directed to recurrent behaviour, as reported by the person, in ordinary real situations. Going beyond this first abstraction, one may decide that the substance of the person's recurrent behaviour can be found in hypothetical or abstract situations which cannot be uniformly referred to real areas of behaviour. Thus one may ask the person what he thinks constitutes a desirable job, or how he thinks children should be brought up. Whether or not his answers can be taken as referring directly to his own job, or to his future family, is arguable. This kind of transferability is even more arguable with the last degree of abstraction, in which one expects to find the substance of the person's recurrent behaviour reflected in what he does in constructed situations (tests, laboratory experiments and so on) that have no analogue at all in ordinary behaviour. The detailed argument may be left to Chapter 9, but it may be noted that the general case for substantial abstraction is strong. Obviously it is economical; if, as has long been the implicit hope of psychology, one can really get at the substance of the person's tediously complex behaviour in a few tests, common experience will not be in the race with psychology. Besides this, there are likely advantages, especially in drawing inferences about the person's intentions, in getting him to do something in the present (whether his performance is openly enacted or purely imaginary) instead of relying solely on his not too accurate memory of his possibly poorly understood past.

The third possible economy of procedure, which may be called *synthetic abstraction*, comes after the enquiry proper, in the treatment of results. There are two stages. In the first, the raw data are classified according to a scheme based on theoretical grounds or on previous experience, but not on inspection of the data. For example, the person's answers are rated on scales for various traits or are classified simply as favourable, neutral or unfavourable with regard to each of a set of qualities. In this stage of synthetic abstraction, the assumption is that the substance of the person's answers may be got by compounding it from its elements according to the general rules of psychological chemistry. There may be a further stage of compounding by statistical aggregation, in which variables that have been arranged as conventional numerical series are summed by means of regression weights or factorial weights. Here the assumption is that the substance of the person's answers may be separated from irrelevant or impure additions by analysis. The saving in time of these two synthetic abstractions, as against the point by point comparative analysis of a mass of data, is obvious. Whether or not one can infer (for example) the person's intentions as easily from aggregated variables as one can from relatively unchanged data is a question best considered in Chapter 10, together with instrumental definition.

So far, the nature of psychological enquiry appears to be contradictory. If enquiry is to be economical, it must be more certain of its results, both in their reputability and in their relevance, than is common experience: and it must also get its results more quickly or less laboriously. One kind of economy may be easy. Psychology can meet the need for studying unmanageably large and complex areas of behaviour by specializing, as everyone does in common experience, and taking the areas separately. Economy by using special methods, however, may not be so easy, for instrumental definition, substantial abstraction and synthetic abstraction may be taken to the point where meaning and relevance are lost. It is at least possible that speed may be gained at the cost of precision, so that an economical procedure might be a compromise, depending on the case, between speed and vagueness, or between precision and toil. If this is true, the two kinds of economy are not comparable, as a brief consideration of an illustrative case will show.

The plan of a proposed investigation states the following:

A. Persons who are about to leave school may be differentiated by:

1. Educational level, from leaving at 14 to graduating from university.
2. Social class (father's occupation).
3. Intelligence (test score).
4. Type of home (family organization, sub-divided as required).

B. The persons thus differentiated will differ also in their outlook on jobs:

1. With regard to the kind of job they expect to get, and will enter.
2. With regard to the kind of job they would prefer and might compete for.
3. With regard to the kind of job they dream about if pressed to nominate a fantasy choice.

C. Differences in outlook may be variously related, for the different classes of persons, to their circumstances, including:
   1. The evaluation of work taught or implied in their homes.
   2. Their identification with the values of the home.
   3. Their standing in their peer group at school.
   4. Their preferences among school subjects.
   5. Their knowledge of, and attitude to, the general social evaluation of work.
   6. Their knowledge of jobs (sub-divided by knowledge of kinds of task, of jobs locally available and by the qualities they would like to find in the job they enter).

Now this plan can be called a hypothesis, for all the elements in it can be defined exactly by the operations necessary to examine them. One may propose as a contrast the rigorously scientific hypothesis that for certain persons tested at an officer selection board the relation between final board grades and summed intelligence test scores is best approximated by the equation $Y = ax^n + b$, where Y is grades in rank order (that is, 1 is the highest grade), X is the measure of intelligence and n is greater than 1, but not greater than 2. This is a very different kind of hypothesis in appearance, but not in fact. The first hypothesis set out proposes a number of comparative questions simultaneously, some about who is to be investigated (A1 to A4), some about what they do (B1 to B3) and the remainder (C1 to C6) about when, or under what circumstances, they do it. Persons leaving school at 14, for example, do this or that under specified circumstances, as compared with persons leaving at 18, who do something else: and so on. The second hypothesis proposes only one comparative question: that, for persons and circumstances of testing which can be exactly specified (though in such cases they often are not), persons of high or low intelligence will be rejected by the board and persons of moderate intelligence will be passed. The only question is about what will happen, but of course the hypothesis could be enlarged to take in other comparative questions, about the persons to whom it will happen and the circumstances under which it will happen. But this holds equally for the first hypothesis. It too could be enlarged by putting in more divisions of the main categories, or it could just as well be reduced by suppressing or omitting some divisions. It may well be that the definition of who, what and when in a psychological hypothesis is changed as the investigation proceeds. But this means only that the experimenter who is alert to the complexity of experience changes his mind as he goes along. The empirical status of the hypothesis (that is, its claim to the title) is given in the definition of its terms by the procedures proposed for the enquiry. In this respect, hypotheses of any size or complexity are on the same footing.

It follows that an economy of procedure which is effected by reducing the area of investigation will not affect the status of the hypothesis. With regard to this kind of economy, hypotheses may be ranged by size from component to general in a repeating series. Thus the hypothesis that the occupational preferences (B2 in the illustrative case) of boys leaving school at 14 (part of A1) will be related to their knowledge of jobs and preferences among school subjects (C6 and C4) is a component of the broader hypothesis. But this in turn could be a component of a more general hypothesis about the person's whole occupational history, taking the transition from school to work as one element in this. In such a case the relation between the components and the general hypothesis is one of simple addition. If the original hypothesis is divided through the who-questions (e.g. by studying boys but not girls or primary school leavers but not others), the possibility of making a sound causal analysis is hardly affected, for the data from which intentional perceptions are to be inferred are derived from parts B and C of the hypothesis. In this case the hypothesis about girls is simply added to the hypothesis about boys and no new procedures are required. The case is not quite the same if the hypothesis is divided through the what-questions or the when-questions; for example, by studying job preferences (B2) only or job knowledge (C6) only. If either of these reductions is made and especially if both are made, the hypothesis is suitable for a classificatory, rather than for a causal analysis. A classification of persons (as in A1 to A4) can be related to the observed differences in the elements studied (i.e. B2 and C6 only), but the inference of intentional perceptions will be much harder as most of the relevant data have been omitted. Of course the classificatory hypothesis is quite valid (empirical, operationally defined) in itself. The only difference with this kind of reduction is that the addition of component hypothesis requires special attention to the relations among elements that appear in one hypothesis only. For example, as an alternative to the reduced hypothesis set out above, it may be proposed to investigate differences between persons (A1 to A4, as before), with regard to their occupational expectations (B1 instead of B2) and the influence of their homes (C1 and C2 instead of C6). If these two reduced hypotheses are then combined, it is implied that at the least the relations between B1 and B2 and between C1, C2 and C6 will be studied. It follows that if the results of separate enquiries are to be combined, it will be necessary to include the results of an enquiry (a third one, that is) into these relations. Apart from the usual difficulties of arguing from one population to another, the combination is by simple addition, followed by an inferential causal analysis which, because of the greater breadth of the general hypothesis, may modify the conclusions of the separate investigations.

The case with economies of procedure is different in principle, as may be seen by taking an extreme example. In simplifying the instruments to be used in investigating the school leaver's perception of his future, one replaces lengthy interviews by short self-administering multiple response or check list questionnaires (i.e. in A4 and the whole of C). Besides this instrumental definition, substantial abstraction is introduced by combining C2, C3 and C5 in one scale measure of social adjustment: and synthetic abstraction follows both in the analysis of questionnaire answers and in the factorial aggregation of scales. The hypothesis so proposed can be broken into parts, and the parts will be additive components under the same conditions as before. Findings about parts of the population (A) can be simply added and findings about elements of the persons' outlook and circumstances (B and C) can be added to findings about other elements with the assistance of findings about relations between the elements to be added. The hypothesis, however, is not at all the same as in the first case, as can be seen by repeating part C. What this now states is that differences in outlook (B, described as before, unless statistical aggregation by scaling is used here) may be variously related, for the different classes of persons (A, described much as before), to their statistically aggregated behaviour in certain test situations (C). In so far as the hypothesis now refers to certain remote generalizations about the persons' circumstances, it may be called abstract, in contrast to the real or common hypothesis that refers directly to the persons' circumstances. Of course it is still a valid hypothesis, for its elements can be defined exactly in terms of the test procedures to be used. It is a classificatory and not a causal hypothesis, for the inference of intentional perceptions from factorized scales is, at the least, more difficult than it is from unabstracted material. As a classificatory hypothesis, it is as capable of addition from component to general as is the real or common hypothesis. But the transition from abstract to real, whether between component or between general hypotheses, is not a comparable process. As it depends on the inference of intentional perceptions, and as the material from which this inference must be made is very different in the two cases, movement from the one to the other requires, not addition, but analogical transfer. It requires, that is to say, an interpretation of the abstract hypothesis (or of the findings) which depends on the assumption that generalized and abstracted conventional measures stand for intentional behaviour in an unambiguously identifiable sense. The assumption would be a particular form of the addition axiom discussed in Chapter 3, and it is now clear that this axiom depends, not on simple addition, but on transfer by analogy.

It is the credibility of this axiom, as it applies to various methods of investigation, that is examined in the following chapters. Here it remains only to emphasize the point implied above, that valid hypotheses are or could be proposed about any field of ordinary behaviour. Maybe this is an obvious point, but it must be allowed that hypotheses in psychology are often confined to what has been called abstract behaviour in the argument above; that is, to behaviour which occurs only in the psychologist's office or laboratory. Where hypotheses of this sort are proposed, there may be no apparent intention, and there is often no attempt, to relate them back to behaviour in ordinary life. This is the usual procedure of what is conventionally known as 'experimental psychology', the psychology which both proposes and rigorously tests hypotheses. As Woodworth and Schlosberg put it [73, p. 2], the experimenter tries to control the conditions of observation; hence he can make the event observed occur when he wishes, can repeat his observations and describe them so that others can repeat them, and can systematically vary the conditions of observation.

Now this is merely a description of the comparative method which is common to all the social sciences. It is reduced to the particular experimental form of the natural sciences, in which the experimenter has complete control over his material, but does not differ otherwise from the method of sociology, as described by MacIver [41], or of social anthropology. That the experimenter can make the event observed occur when he wishes is, indeed, peculiar to 'experimental psychology'. That he can repeat his observations, and that he and other workers can repeat them under varying conditions, are commonplaces of the comparative method in any field. Woodworth and Schlosberg, indeed, observe [73, p. 1]: 'that we do not yet know exactly how to subject some of the biggest problems to a rigorous experiment'. It has already been argued that there is no question of the psychologist's being able to subject to control the larger events in which he is immersed. It is therefore difficult to see anything more in this remark than that some psychologists prefer not to undertake the larger and less controllable comparative analyses.

It is a historical curiosity that 'experimental psychology' is still the name of a special branch of study. The similar specialization of 'social psychology' is possible because the study of the isolated individual is at least conceivable. The non-empirical study of psychology is inconceivable; so that any psychology which proceeds by sound comparative analyses (as all psychological enquiry does) is entitled to be called experimental. The point is emphasized because control of the matter of investigation is only one, and not necessarily the most important one, of the conditions of sound experimental procedure. Asking questions that are appropriate to the hypothesis is an essential first step; laying out the procedure so that the simple multivariate analysis of the natural sciences can be applied to the results cannot be a first step and may not be appropriate at all. 'Experimental' procedures, in the narrow sense, are not specially referred to in the following discussion because it is not their technical detail that matters. If one starts with the possibility of investigating hypotheses about any field of ordinary behaviour, what matters is how a compromise is to be reached in using economical but relevant methods. This requires the consideration, not of 'experimental' procedures as such, but of the assumptions upon which they are based; or rather of the processes by which they are built up. The rigorously scientific 'experimenter' devises as a matter of course methods of investigation which do not bear on ordinary behaviour, which narrowly prescribe the person's response and which yield quasi-physical measures that can be treated by elaborate statistical methods. The 'experimenter', that is to say, puts his methods through the processes of substantial abstraction and instrumental definition before he begins work, and applies categorical and statistical abstraction (together, synthetic abstraction) to the data that he collects. These processes are used as a matter of course, but are none the less deliberate. As it is their effects that have to be considered, it is these processes that need discussion (and hence naming, for the purpose of discussion) before the status of the addition (or analogical transfer) axiom can be considered.

At this point it is sufficient to observe that analogical transfer is not comparable to addition, and to leave the discussion of its validity to the following chapters, including Chapter 12, where its implications with regard to the nature of law in psychology are discussed. It may be worth noting, however, that the distinction drawn is not peculiar to psychology. An analogy is found in the work of the zoologist, who may study all the characteristics of a species, genus and so on, or who may specialize in the comparative study of single organs or processes, such as the primate skull or the chemistry of vertebrate skeletal muscle. If comparative morphology had been undertaken before taxonomy, the effect on the development of zoology would have been interesting. The study of history provides a closer analogy. The study of the development of whole societies is general and causal. The sociological study of the present organization of societies is a component study, in so far as it is a-historical and therefore tends to be classificatory rather than causal. The study of smaller and smaller elements in the development of a society (from political history taken by itself through to the history of single institutions such as the school and single artefacts such as the chair), proceeds from real and causal studies to abstract and classificatory. It is again interesting to speculate how history would have developed if it has begun with the monograph topics.

SUBSTANTIAL ABSTRACTION IN METHODS OF ENQUIRY

THE detailed discussion of methods is best begun with substantial abstraction for, if this is done, it is the first and chief process involved in the selection of methods. The psychologist decides first what kind of general methods to use (e.g. whether to use interviews, aptitude tests or psychological measurements) and then decides how to treat his results. The internal arrangement of his methods, which may involve instrumental definition, comes into the first decision, but only as a subsidiary question, and is therefore better treated together with synthetic abstraction.

Methods generally may be said to range in structure from those that put the person into something closely similar to a real life situation to those that put him into a specially constructed situation with no counterpart in ordinary life. This range must be considered from the point of view of economy of use. For convenience, it will be assumed that all methods are concerned with present behaviour and especially with recurrent behaviour, or at least with behaviour that could be repeated. Within these limits, economy must be considered with regard to both speed and precision and especially with regard to the possible contradiction between these two requirements. This will involve the consideration of the areas of behaviour to which the kinds of method can be applied, or are usually applied; and also the consideration of the extent to which the person's intentional perceptions can be inferred from the data and to which findings can be transferred to apparently similar cases. Lastly, it will be necessary to note what least degree of instrumental definition is necessary for each kind of method, for no method can work without some degree of definition.

Group 1. *Ordinary sustained acquaintance*

This may be taken as a method for the sake of contrast, as its inadequacy is the reason for the existence of psychology. Strictly defined, it includes only knowing the person in ordinary situations in which one is engaged with him for some common purpose other than that of knowing him; but this definition would include the psychologist's incidental use of such non-professional knowledge, if he is willing to use it. However, even in this very limited respect the method is doubtfully economical. That it is the most laborious method is obvious but, besides that, its precision is open to doubt in so far as its usefulness depends on sufficient acquaintance in a close personal relation. It might be argued that such close acquaintance is the only way of knowing covert behaviour, of understanding someone else by the analogical reconstruction of his experience. So far as this is true, real acquaintance gives more possibility of a sound intentional analysis than any special method can; but here again its precision may be greatly reduced by emotional involvement, as may the transferability of understood experience from one person to another. Its one advantage is that, being continuous and spontaneous, it needs, and indeed is capable of, no definition. As a method of psychological enquiry, then, real acquaintance can hardly be more than an occasional accessory; though of course its rejection in this special field does not touch its position as the method of practical understanding of other persons or of oneself. For this purpose it is the special methods that are occasional accessories.

Group 2. *Observation and the biographical interview*

This is not a method but a broad group of methods, the common characteristic of which is that they all refer directly to the person's present actual behaviour. The group includes observation of ordinary behaviour, but not of specially enacted behaviour. Thus participant research is placed here if it involves only participation in some common action other than psychological training or learning; otherwise it goes into group 3, or overlaps both groups. The ordinary observation of behaviour (in the classroom, playground, factory and so on) is included in group 2. So are interview methods which invite the person to talk about things as they are or were, over the whole range of actual behaviour. Interviewing the person about his habitual overt behaviour in any field, about particular events in his effective present, about his occasional symbolic behaviour, whether overt or covert (e.g. his opinions, attitudes and ideology), and about any other kind of covert behaviour that he can report (e.g. his aspirations, goals, daydreams, fears and anxieties), are all included here. The

111

biographical interview is therefore to be understood in a broad sense, though biography in the strict sense is not excluded: the person's report of his past behaviour of any of the kinds mentioned (that is, of his present past) belongs here too.

This group of methods therefore includes a wide variety of established procedures. Besides the observation procedures already mentioned, the clinical interview, the employment interview, the vocational guidance interview and the interview conducted for general research purposes (on any scale from opinion polling up) all belong to this group, and so do psychoanalysis and group therapy. The methods in this group could be said to depend on condensed acquaintance: knowing the person in real life over some years is replaced by knowing him over a few days or hours (when he is observed) or at second hand, over an even shorter time (when he is interviewed). It must be allowed, of course, that an element of pure enactment, or projective construction, may come into an interview even if it is apparently directed only to matters of fact. The person does not necessarily have an opinion on all the matters about which the psychologist asks his opinion, but he may none the less oblige by producing one: and, depending on how he sees his part as a person being interviewed by an expert, he may colour the reporting of overt behaviour in the way that he thinks is expected. So far as such things happen in the interview, it must be grouped with the openly projective methods, especially those of group 4. Besides this, interviewing is necessarily limited to matters which the person can articulate and is willing to report. It is a method of very general applicability, but is limited in any area of behaviour by the person's verbal sophistication and is therefore particularly limited in investigating complex symbolic behaviour. Covert behaviour that the person does not wish to report, or cannot report, is obviously inaccessible, except in psychoanalysis.

The methods of group 2 are time consuming even if, as a limiting case, a questionnaire is substituted for the interview; but they are on the whole economical on account of the amount and variety of information that they gather if properly handled. It is necessary, of course, to strike a practical compromise between the short stereotyped interview and the interview in which the person is asked every possible question, regardless of his interest. Both interviewing and observation, however, have what the mental testers would call high face validity. In most circumstances it is easy (it may even be too easy) to get the co-operation of the persons to be interviewed. All that seems to be necessary for this is to explain how the purpose of the interview is relevant to some of the person's purposes; and many persons will accept the interview as relevant even if it is being done solely in order to advance knowledge. On the other hand, the acceptability of the interview may be much lower where it is directly concerned with the solution of practical problems. Persons who have a somewhat crude idea of the scientific nature of psychology may rather object to the counselling interview, and still more to the therapeutic interview (both of which are forms of participant research) and may even object to interviewing as a means of surveying a problem (e.g. of industrial morale). Where the person wants something out of the psychologist's magic box, interviewing is not economical: it is just not possible unless the ground can be prepared for it. The same holds for observation methods generally, and it may be noted that the device of observing in disguise (which is sometimes used even where open observing would be accepted) seems also to be uneconomical. Apart from the possibility of unpleasant repercussions, which need not be considered here, this device ensures acceptability at the cost of severe restriction in the observer's scope and this kind of condensed acquaintance is not obviously worth much.

Economy in the sense of precision is more certain. The methods of group 2 take the person's real life behaviour directly as it is. Subject only to the reservations made above about the person's possible unwillingness or inability to report his behaviour as it is, these methods are therefore eminently suited for the inference of intentions. Further, if the data are reasonably extensive, findings can be transferred from observed or reported situations to similar situations with a fair degree of confidence.

These methods are also easy to use in that they require little definition. A check list of the kinds of behaviour to be observed or of the areas to be explored in the interview, perhaps with some probing questions, is the least degree of definition that is necessary and it is sufficient for most purposes.

Groups 3 to 6. Projective methods generally

These four groups include methods that, by contrast with those of group 2, are indirect. They put the person in situations that are vaguely or sharply defined and that are all imaginable as real life situations. The less abstract may be taken by the person to refer to situations he knows, while the more abstract he can only refer to an imaginary inner situation. The more abstract methods, of course, are real in the same sense as the interview; they are concerned with the person's aspirations, fantasies, attitudes and perhaps his habits in the present test situation, while the interview is concerned with the same kinds of behaviour in a situation which, strictly considered, is also removed from reality or ordinary experience. However, this logical resemblance is less important than the fact that the interview is, as far as possible, directed to actual past experience; in this respect the less abstract projective methods, which can perhaps be referred to actual experience, are more similar to the methods of group 2, and indeed overlap with them. The groups of projective methods are discussed in rank order of abstraction, though this order is not so clear cut as the numbering may suggest.

Group 3. *The staged situation*

In this group of methods the psychologist describes a situation which the persons are required to enact. The methods vary somewhat in their structure and purpose and hence in their degree of abstraction, but all use situations that could reasonably be (and therefore may be) within the experience of the persons concerned. The group includes participant discussion methods as described by Jaques [30] that are used deliberately for the purpose of training in the conduct of affairs as well as for immediately practical purposes. It also includes the psychodrama, as it is used by Maier [43] in human relations training. These methods, which are designed for action rather than for research, could be classed in group 2 in so far as they use situations that have occurred or are actually going on. However, the element of deliberate re-enactment or of double role-playing distinguishes them from this group, even though the distinction is by no means sharp. Other role-playing methods, whether they are used primarily for general research or for practical purposes such as selection, clearly belong in this group so long as they present a realistic and imaginable situation. Thus the range of methods includes group discussions on topics of general interest, psychodramas with real life characters, and group planning or other group tasks in which the material presented is taken from real life though not necessarily from the actual field of experience of the persons concerned. No precise line can be drawn between these methods and the more fantastic (that is, more abstract) methods that are classed in group 6, but the extreme cases that would obviously belong to this latter group would be discussions on esoteric topics, psychodramas with comic strip characters and group tasks with material taken from melodramatic thrillers.

In principle, group 3 could include test situations enacted by one person alone, but these are better placed elsewhere. Problem-solving tests, for example, may include questions that are drawn from ordinary experience, and it could even be said that intelligence tests which include verbal syllogisms and number series (but not diagrammatic items) draw on ordinary experience. However, it seems doubtful that this kind of generalized and fragmentary conceptual experience is relevant, as it is subsidiary to all the areas of behaviour described in Chapter 8 and its only analogue in real life is the school examination. These tests are therefore placed in group 8. The case with psychomotor tests is different. Many of these resemble nothing but themselves, but some are exact imitations of actual work tasks, and these certainly require the enactment of a real situation. However, tests of this latter kind are used only in selection for and training in quite complicated tasks. When they are used in selection, they are probably so strange to the person who has never seen the task before that they are better classified with the other motor tests, in group 9. Used in training by a person who has some practice in the task, they are a special case of observation in real life, which belongs in group 2. It follows that the methods of group 3 are chiefly applicable to social behaviour, though conceptual behaviour (planning and arguing) and even the incidental handling of things may usefully be observed at the same time.

These methods are not very economical in one sense, in that they are tedious to arrange or to construct and to conduct. Further, except in participant work, where recording is usually impossible, making a reasonably full record of proceedings is very difficult. They are fairly acceptable to the persons chosen as actors but sometimes less so to other persons who may want role-playing methods used for practical purposes (such as selection) and whose understanding of the magic box procedure may lead them to expect fantastic situations. Economy in the sense of precision is unfortunately unknown. The few empirical studies that have been made of the validity of role-playing procedures in selection show that there is not much relation between assessments of performance and final assessments based on wider evidence. This suggests that in these procedures the supposed analogy between the enacted situation and performance in the task for which persons are being selected is not at all close. However, experience of role-playing methods suggests that this is not so with well-devised situations. In the real life case of Jaques [30] or the enacted real cases of Maier [43] it is clear enough, if only by common sense inspection of the records or by observation of the acting, that the person's intentions in the enacted situation can be inferred unambiguously and in some detail. The only condition under which this is not possible is if the person does not get into the part and so acts badly, not developing the role in his own terms, but trying out and dropping successive possibilities; but this, which may derive from poor construction of the situation, is obvious enough when it happens.

However, the transfer of inferences made in the enacted situation to other situations is an entirely open question. It should be possible with a high degree of confidence and in considerable detail, if the real situations are closely similar to those enacted and if the inferences made can be fairly generalized; that is, can be taken beyond the person's present intentions to include his habits and general goals. Neither analogy nor the possibility of generalization has been explored at all, so that the methods of this group cannot yet be regarded as having fulfilled their apparent promise of precision.

For much the same reason, the least degree of definition necessary for these methods to work cannot be exactly stated. It is clear that the situation must be described in some detail and that factual descriptions are more effective than atmospheric (e.g. one states what X did or said rather than what kind of person he is); and it seems that the best situation (apart from series of real situations) is one that can be enacted in an hour to an hour and a half. However, these features of organization also remain to be investigated.

Group 4. The hypothetical situation

This group includes interview and questionnaire methods that present the person with a conceptual situation that he can understand as it is presented whether or not it is in his past experience. The questions asked invite him to report his opinions, attitudes, intentions or aspirations after making a comparative analysis that he has probably not made before. The whole group of methods is experimental in that the person is told how to conduct an experiment on himself and report the results, but what he uses in the experiment is his concepts of real events that he can imagine if he has not experienced them. These methods are very useful in extending the ordinary interview into inner personal areas which are beyond its reach because the person lacks the verbal sophistication or, more particularly, the conceptual articulation necessary to respond to direct questions. The hypothetical situation gives him something that he can articulate on the spot: it systematizes the fluid disorder of his half-formed ideas. These methods may also be useful in getting opinions that the person is unwilling to refer to a real situation but is prepared to refer to a hypothetical one. While the methods are chiefly of use in exploring conceptual behaviour, and especially in exploring that part of it which is not normally overt (that is, in exploring the most important part of the person's self-directed activities), they may be of considerable use in other areas in so far as it can be inferred that the person has referred the hypothetical situation to his actual past experience and is indirectly reporting real events.

As these methods are a special extension of the ordinary interview and not full scale methods by themselves, a number of particular examples may be given.

(*a*) An adaptation of the Bavelas questionnaire on good and bad things to do was used by Oeser and Hammond [50, Ch. 14] and Oeser and Emery [51, Ch. 8] to investigate the home behaviour of groups of Australian children. The results show clearly the child's perception of the values of his parents, which even a sophisticated adult would have difficulty in reporting in answer to a direct question. There is also a good deal of information on what the child actually does at home, for it can reasonably be supposed that most, if not all, of the activities he reports as things for which he is praised or blamed are things he has done.

(*b*) In one of these investigations (Oeser and Hammond, [50, Ch. 8]), the question: 'what should a man's main aims in life be?' was asked to test the relative importance in the person's life of his family, his work and other activities. This was extended, in an industrial enquiry conducted by the author (the analysis of which is in progress), into a set of comparisons in which the person decides what he would do in a situation where his work and family interests, or his personal and class interests, and so on, are in conflict. Both the general form (which is the more effective) and the detailed form show clearly how the person stands with regard to the conventional values of his society, at least as far as family affairs and work are concerned. It is not so clear that these methods give any indirect information about overt behaviour, for a person can easily put his job before his family, his family or friends before his society, and so on, in abstract evaluation but reverse the order in practice. However, it may be supposed that there is some relation between evaluation and practice.

(*c*) The question: 'can you think of anything you would like to change in the factory?' was included in the interview check list used in the industrial enquiry referred to under (*b*). If the person interviewed has made any criticisms of the factory, the answers to this question discriminate their importance to him more clearly than a direct question would. For example, if he criticizes the lighting and ventilation but does not suggest changing them, it can be assumed that he is not seriously aggrieved by them; or if he criticizes his foreman at length and briefly remarks that his pay is insufficient, and then says that the pay is the only thing he would like to change, it is probably that pay is his source of grievance. Further, the person may mention features he would like to change without having previously made any criticisms and one may then be able to infer how he perceives his work in relation to his other activities. If he says, for example, that there should be provision for job transfers because the work is monotonous, it is likely that the job is 'ust a job to him (though he might well be unable to put it so simply in answer to a direct question) and that the centre of his interests is outside work.

(*d*) The hypothetical question is used to assist diagnosis in the clinical interview. For example, if there is doubt whether the person's headaches and stomach pains are due to his having too difficult a job (as he says) or are due to his frustrated ambition or to some combination of these factors, he may be asked what he would do if he were offered, or if he had to take over for a time, the next job above his. His answer should show clearly how he perceives the status of his job in relation to his evaluation of himself, especially as he is likely to refer the hypothetical question directly to his present situation. In this case the question gives him a direct lead through the tangle of his blocked perceptions.

(*e*) A question that has been fairly widely used is; 'what would be the best/the worst thing that could happen to you?' These do not so much refer to a particular hypothetical situation as invite the person to select the appropriate situations. If the questions are asked in context, in the course of a biographical interview and paired with questions about the best and worst things that have happened, they are quite effective in eliciting hopes and fears that are too inarticulate, too private or even too fantastic to be reported in response to a more direct question.

(*f*) The opinion poll sets a hypothetical situation if it refers to remote possibilities, as when the person is asked whether he approves or disapproves the idea of higher education for aborigines. A question like this, in the same way as the more elaborate questions of social attitude scales, pins the person down to evaluating a specified situation, where he might be unable to make an articulate report of his attitude if he were asked an open general question. What he reports, of course, is his perception of a possibility: as Sherif [61, Ch. 10] stresses, if he were presented with the fact instead, his attitude might be different.

(*g*) A more elaborate example of the use of the hypothetical situation to press the person to make an evaluation may be taken from the investigation of job preferences referred to in Chapter 7. This was carried out in a town in which there was very heavy unemployment, so that the school leavers concerned in it expressed job preferences and expectations, in response to direct questions, that were realistic and unambitious. Making paired comparisons through a list of jobs that included some beyond all but their wildest dreams enabled them to make an indirect report of these dreams.

The list of examples could be extended indefinitely, as the hypothetical question is the natural and critically important extension of the biographical interview. The examples given are sufficient to demonstrate the common feature of the methods of this group: they all invite the person to make a comparative analysis of material which is within the scope of his imagination. If the question put is beyond the imagination of most persons (e.g.: 'what would you do if you didn't have to work at all?'), it belongs to group 6, the most abstract projective methods. In the same way, questions put in the biographical interview may belong here rather than in group 2 if they invite an imaginative projection: for example, a question about how the person likes his boss may require imaginative projection rather than a report of present fact if he hardly knows his boss. As no sharp delimitation of group 4 is possible, the efficiency of any particular method as a projective method depends on the definition of the situation. The least degree of definition necessary is that which will enable the person to imagine the situation put, while definition beyond this degree (as, for example, in the elaboration of possible best and worst things, in case (e), above) may force him back irrelevantly to his actual experience. However, the question of definition can only be settled empirically.

The methods of this group are economical in the simple sense in the same way as the biographical interview when they are part of this and are equally economical (fast in use, acceptable) when they are more like special test methods. Their precision is high for, if they are well designed, they are bound to give data from which intentional perceptions can be inferred. This is their purpose, to push beyond matters of fact into matters of intention. However, the transferability of findings is more contentious. That findings can be transferred to closely analogous situations may be assumed: but the methods of group 4 depend on the presenting of a hypothetical situation. It may be reasonable to assume transfer to similar hypothetical situations, so that some stability of perception can be assumed (e.g. the person who perceives chronic illness as the worst thing that could happen to him will go on worrying about his health). It may also be reasonable to assume some degree of stability in another sense, in the transfer of findings from one population to equivalent groups (e.g. from primary school leavers in one place to primary school leavers generally). It is not at all clear, however, that findings can be transferred from the hypothetical to the actual situation. For example, the person who does suffer chronic illness may not be at all overcome by his misfortune and the man who has been a process worker for many years may no longer perceive any attractions in the artisan's or the doctor's jobs (though data from the industrial enquiry mentioned above indicate that in this case there is quite a high degree of stability). The point is that in the progress of substantial abstraction, the methods of group 4 are the first (if one accepts those of group 3 as depending on real situations) that abstract from and generalize ordinary behaviour. This is therefore the first group for which transferability in the sense described cannot be assumed on the strength of a possibly rather remote analogy, but must be determined empirically.

Group 5. Contextless projective tests

This group includes all the methods that are usually called projective tests, which are next in order of abstraction because it is difficult or impossible to relate the test situation to any real public situation. The Picture-Frustration Test is perhaps the most definite of the well-known tests, but it has hardly more than a comic strip resemblance to reality. The Thematic Apperception Test is more abstract because of the deliberate vagueness of its pictures as well as the fantastic nature of some. Sentence-completion and word-association tests may have fragmentary and accidental links with ordinary behaviour, and the Rorschach Test does not have even these. However, if the situations that these tests present are not of a kind that the person can refer to his or anybody else's overt behaviour, they are such that he may be able to refer them directly to his covert behaviour and especially to his fantasies. Thus the Picture-Frustration Test presents situations similar to frustrations he has brooded over and the Thematic Apperception Test situations similar to his more sustained (and more private, or even unconscious) compensatory or abreactive fantasies. Sentence-completion and word-association Tests invite him to repeat some of his fleeting, hardly formulated and perhaps incongruous ideas and associations and the Rorschach test invites him to enact his very vaguest fantasies, as when he sees pictures in the fire or on the wall. These tests have no context in that they are quite remote from overt behaviour, but if they do refer directly to the person's ordinary covert fantasy behaviour they are no more abstract than the methods of group 3.

Their placing, however, must depend on the systematic investigation of their general economy, which unfortunately has hardly been attempted. It can be said that they are fairly easy to make (a point which is relevant for the first time with this group, as systematic test construction begins here) and are quick to use and acceptable to the persons tested. Besides the test material itself, the only definition they require is that given by a form of introduction which is sufficient to get the person interested: definition beyond this minimum degree (e.g. by suggesting what to look for in the pictures or the inkblots) gives short and stereotyped responses. These tests, then, are economical in their application. Their precision, however, has been almost entirely unexplored, either by the psychologists who use them or by those who deplore their use. A projective test would be precise in the general sense, if besides getting repeatable results (which can be assumed), it got results capable of some general applicability. It is not designed, of course, to elicit behaviour from which intentional perceptions can be inferred, but is designed to elicit what might be called sub-intentional behaviour, including the whole range of covert behaviour that the person cannot report directly, from that which is merely too fragmentary and inarticulate to report through accessible matters that the person might not care to report to, in some degree, the inaccessible repressed. One can perhaps assume that the projective test, like all tests and indeed all procedures of any kind, to some extent, does penetrate to the fragmentary and obscure sub-intentional ground of the person's articulate behaviour, both overt and covert. But one has to ask the difficult question, in what sense is this the ground of articulate behaviour? What is the relation between the obscure, thus explored, and the open or articulate? It may be assumed that the results of projective tests could be transferred to equivalent populations, but this means only that there is some consistency between persons in the obscure grounds explored, in the same way as repeatability depends on consistency from time to time.

The critical question, however, is that of consistency between situations and, at this degree of substantial abstraction, no simple assumption of analogy will suffice to answer the question. The possibility of transferring findings to real situations (the only transfer that matters) depends on two factors. It is necessary to generalize the organization of the person's sub-intentional behaviour from the results of a test or of several tests; to say, that is, that his present actual fantasies (not only his fantasies in the test situation) have describable components, the relations among which can be stated. Then it is necessary to know just how this organized, but not directly accessible, behaviour is related to accessible behaviour in real situations. The clinical use of projective tests touches neither of these problems. The empathic and intuitive judgement is doubtless sound for the purpose for which it is used but, because it places immediate practical applicability before communicability, it makes an unanalysed impressionistic generalization and assumes a direct transfer to real situations. The problems raised can be answered only by a detailed internal analysis of projective tests, followed by an analysis of the relations between tests (and, incidentally, between testers) and then by an analysis of the relations between tests and findings of various kinds about real behaviour. It is important to note that this last analysis cannot be only a statistical study of the test's validity, or forecasting efficiency. Studies of this kind, as discussed by Cronbach [15, Ch. 20) show what the test does, but may not show at all how it does it, and this information is necessary. The transfer of sub-intentional behaviour, as generalized in the first two analyses, to real situations requires that one should be able to trace the correspondences and differences, point by point, between articulate behaviour and its ground.

In view of the wide use and equally wide misunderstanding of projective tests, it is relevant to give some actual findings for two tests that were used by the author in an officer selection board. One of these was a reduction of the Thematic Apperception Test, in which the group of persons tested wrote stories about seven selected pictures. The stories that a sample wrote about the first picture (6 BM in the original test: often known as 'Mother and Son') were classified under four general themes: the son is going out to make his way in the world, is a bad lot, is thinking of getting married, and lastly various family dramas including father, sibs and strangers as well as, or instead of, the son. Within each of these themes, the stories were classified under three outcomes: obstacles are overcome and all ends well, there is no conclusion to the story, and all ends miserably, the son and perhaps others going from bad to worse. This classification was compared with two judgements made during the course of the board's work, the general diagnosis made by the psychiatrist and the board's final assessment of the person's potential as an officer. These judgements depended very little, even indirectly, on the projective test material and were substantially independent of each other: the only significant relation observed is that an excessive proportion of persons diagnosed as hysteric or as having anxiety states was rejected by the board and for this relation the coefficient of association, phi, is only 0.30. All differential findings reported below are significant at or beyond this level (P less than 0.01).

It is found that persons diagnosed as normal prefer the 'bad lot' theme, the compulsives and schizoid characters prefer the 'marriage drama' and the hysterics and other anxious persons prefer the other two themes: the son makes good, and the mixed family drama. The classification by outcomes is even simpler: the three groups of persons prefer happy endings, no endings and general disaster respectively. This generalization from one story suggests that what the diagnostic classification does is to separate the normal persons who can cope with the ordinary ups and downs of life from the rigid persons who cannot cope but who try to bend life to suit their ways and from the anxious who are terrified of life. The leap from sub-intentional behaviour (or the handling of fantasies) to behaviour in real situations in general is considerable and cannot, of course, be made on such slight evidence. But this analysis shows the way in which the first part of the evidence (analysis of the psychiatrist's diagnosis, as of behaviour in general, requires separate consideration) should be gathered, and the next step can be demonstrated in principle by considering the relations of the other judgement, the board's final grade, to the classification of stories.

These relations are not so systematic, as themes and outcomes are confounded. It is found that persons graded as acceptable wrote either stories in which the hero triumphed over odds or cynical stories in which he went from bad to worse; persons graded as possible wrote either conventional stories in which the hero makes good against no great odds or inconclusive stories; and the unacceptable persons wrote either vague or miserable stories. This rather suggests a classification of the persons tested into the bold, the cautious and the hopeless. Here again, this generalization and implied transfer need backing up by much more evidence, from the analysis of the other six stories as well as the analysis of the stories in relation to other judgements and other kinds of behaviour. However, the second step is correctly made even if it is only a small step, and a third may be demonstrated by considering some results of the word-association test.

In this, the persons tested were required to write down the first thing they thought of, whether words, phrases or sentences, as a series of words on cards was exposed to them at the rate of four a minute. The results set out are selected from the most valid found in the trial analysis of the first five words in a total list of fifty.

It is found that responses to the word 'book' (the second word shown) are related to the psychiatrist's diagnosis in this way: normal persons make brief and vague responses, or write clichés (e.g. 'reading good', 'read inwardly and digest'), compulsives and schizoid characters make rather highbrow general expository responses (e.g. 'like technical subjects', 'Books library and book tokens'), and anxious persons make responses with a personal reference (e.g. 'I like reading', 'I could read a book now'). For what it is worth, this suggests some parallel to the classification into those who can cope normally (in this case, with a trivial subject), those whose habits are inflexible and those who cannot cope, in that even a harmless word is taken personally. There are suggestive parallels also in the relations between board gradings and responses to the words 'beer' (the first shown) and 'break' (the third shown). Persons accepted by the board tended to make brisk, definite and impersonal responses to both words, persons regarded as doubtful tended to make definite responses with a personal reference, and the unacceptable tended to clichés, evasions or no response. In both these cases there is some ground for expecting generalization from test to test.

It is not suggested, of course, that these few and briefly reported results are of any real use in establishing the transferability of findings from the conventional projective tests that are included in group 5. However, they do go far enough beyond the mere assertion that transferability should be investigated to show both that it can be investigated by the conventional methods of comparative analysis, and that the investigation is promising. It is important that these things should be shown, for the clinical psychologist's practical use of projective tests gives no more ground for asserting transferability than the empiricists' mistaken ideas of how these tests work do for denying it. If these two schools had said all that could be said about projective tests, the tests would have to be abandoned as a general method of psychological enquiry, which would be at the least unfortunate, as no other method proposes to penetrate to sub-intentional behaviour in a short time. Meantime, the tests may be classed as group 5 on the conservative ground that their degree of substantial abstraction cannot be stated definitely but may be high.

Group 6. Projective methods with a fantasy context

As any method of enquiry may to some extent require projective behaviour on the part of the persons being examined it might be expected that projective tests other than the well-known contextless kind would require consideration. Included in this group, therefore, are the remaining indirect methods of enquiry. These are methods that present a situation which, if it is very hard to imagine, is not inconceivable in real life. Superficially, therefore, these methods are less abstract than those of group 5, which present a possible situation (beyond the secondary presentation of the test situation itself, as in all methods) only in so far as they relate directly to the person's actual or imaginable sub-intentional behaviour. However, the methods of group 6 are regarded as having the higher degree of substantial abstraction because they are not capable of direct reference either to the person's overt behaviour or to his covert behaviour. They are too fantastic or too elaborate to work in the way that other indirect tests do: which amounts to saying that this group includes only inefficient tests.

This is true, for example, of some tests that might belong to group 3 if they were more realistic. A group discussion on the meaning of happiness, for example, may be quite without the scope of senior civil servants, but it would certainly baffle a group of foremen. The wide variety of group tasks (leaderless, both physical and planning, and with an appointed leader) with sketchy and highly melodramatic plots that was used in war time officer selection procedures probably belongs in this group for the most part. The apparent principle of construction of most of them was to include as much violent action or imaginary violence as possible. If this presents a situation which can be imagined (which one may doubt) it certainly does not present one that could reasonably be within the experience of the persons tested: for the testing programme was introduced as a substitute for knowledge of what the person had done in action. The same kind of doubt attaches to individual tests of the person's practical ingenuity, of the kind which required him to manœuvre some awkward object over an obstacle course that might be as much imaginary as visible and that was not meant to be credible. The doubt is strongest with individual tests of physical capacity (or endurance or toughness or courage), in which the person was required to do acrobatic feats on ropes, ladders, trees, poles and so on. Though this procedure obviously has considerable shop window value, it does not appear that it bears even the remotest relation to the person's ordinary behaviour.

These procedures are at once too fantastic to be referred to the person's ordinary behaviour, for presenting him with imaginary minefields, tanks, chasms and fences means stretching his imagination beyond the breaking point; and too elaborate to be referred to his fantasy behaviour, for the elaboration of quasi-real detail prevents him from shaping the situation at all freely. There are other probably inefficient methods that have only one of these weaknesses. Asking the person, for example, what he would do if he had no need to work at all, or what he would do if he won a million pounds in a lottery, is rather likely to elicit a vague or stereotyped response only, or none. This is too fantastic to be related to his aspirations or articulate daydreams; if it were not, it would belong in group 4, with questions which can be so related. An example of the weakness of over-elaboration is a projective test of the ordinary sort (that is, belonging to group 5 in principle) that was used in the early stages of the industrial enquiry referred to previously in this chapter. It was thought that, as unsophisticated persons have difficulty with projective tests requiring considerable verbal fluency, they would be more at home with a story-completion test that did nine-tenths of the work for them, leaving them only the conclusion to draw. This was a move in the wrong direction. The test obtained little more than a few common stereotyped responses because it assisted the person to the point at which he had very little freedom of movement.

Whether or not the procedures described are inefficient could only be shown, of course, by a full analysis and until this is done the question of their placing remains open. One possibility is that they would be found to be as efficient as the tests they resemble or modifiable so as to be equally efficient; and in this case they would be classed in other groups. Or they might be found to be irretrievably inefficient and would then be abandoned. The third possibility is that they would be found to be efficient enough to retain in use, as they are or modified, but efficient in their own way. It is possible, for example, that the fantasy-enactment procedures described do get at some mixture of intentional behaviour that could be transferred to real situations and sub-intentional behaviour that could be generalized as the ground of behaviour in real situations: which would be a compound of groups 3 and 5. It is also possible that a story-completion test, properly handled, would produce a compound like this. While these possibilities are open, it is as well to retain a distinct group in the general array of methods against the time when the matter has been determined.

Group 6, then, might be regarded as a ragbag of tests that are not abstract enough to classify with the abstract tests but too abstract to classify with the other indirect procedures.

Groups 7 to 9. Particulate tests generally

The indirect methods of groups 3 to 6 differ sufficiently in their degree of substantial abstraction to be rankable in order. They differ more, however, in their fields of application, from real behaviour which can be enacted or analysed to the sub-intentional or intellectual grounds of overt behaviour. These methods therefore differ on the common basis of their being indirect, of their referring to behaviour which is at least imaginable if it cannot be actually reinstated: and this common basis is in turn the ground for expecting that the findings of these methods should be capable of some transfer to real situations, beyond what transfer has been investigated and is known to be possible.

The methods of enquiry that remain to be discussed include all personality tests of the inventory type, interest inventories, adjustment questionnaires, trait rating schemes and so on; and all tests of intelligence, special abilities, aptitudes and scholastic achievements; and lastly, all tests of motor skills. This collection of methods thus includes the whole range of tests in the usual sense or, more precisely, the whole range of particulate tests; that is, tests consisting of a number of small and unconnected items or of a number of repetitions of the one small item. The methods in groups 7 to 9 differ sufficiently among themselves for the groups to need distinguishing, but here again the differences in rank order are less important than the common feature of all groups, which is the abstract nature of the test material. In this respect these methods, if they are rankable in order after the indirect methods, differ almost as markedly from these latter as they do from the methods of observation and interviewing, in group 2. From indirect to abstract methods is not so much another step as a sudden leap.

This may be shown by considering in what sense particulate tests are abstract. The situations they present are abstract in that it is very hard, if not impossible, for the person tested even to imagine them occurring in reality, let alone to reinstate his previous experience of such situations. His real behaviour bears no conceivable resemblance to the behaviour required of him in the test. At all events, this is true of his ordinary connected behaviour; that is, behaviour in ordinary areas or covert behaviour backing this up, and recurrent behaviour with an appreciable duration. It may not be true of the person's fragmentary behaviour. He may be able to find an analogy with the test situation in his simplest and most superficial opinions or attitudes, in the smallest elements of his general knowledge and in his daily motor activities. So far as this analogy is at least imaginable, the particulate tests could be regarded as indirect methods of exploring overt fragmentary behaviour in all fields. However, if the reference to fragmentary behaviour is possible, it is irrelevant because it is never made. Not even the most compulsive person would make it for himself in the test situations and the psychologist naturally does not make it because he uses particulate tests as a quick means of exploring the substance of the person's real behaviour. He expects the results of these methods to be transferable not to fragmentary but to ordinary connected behaviour, whether overt, intellectual or sub-intentional. Now this transfer would depend, not on analogy between real and test behaviour, but on the addition of fragments of test behaviour to make real behaviour, which is a new and radically different process. The efficiency of particulate tests depends chiefly on the validity of particular forms of the addition axiom and these will therefore be discussed for each of the three groups separately. The economy in use of all particulate tests may be disposed of generally, as it is the chief reason for the popularity of these tests. All are relatively easy to construct and validate, and most are easy to administer and score, though this is not so true of psychomotor tests, which must usually be given individually and may be a little tedious to score. It may be noted that validation and scoring are facilitated by the very common practice of constructing tests in groups 7 and 8 with forced choice answers. This degree of definition is not strictly necessary to the test's operation, but the use of open problems with creative answers would not affect the general argument. Finally, all particulate tests are acceptable; they are so well established that the persons being tested or the persons for whom the testing is being done may be baffled if they are not used.

Group 7. *Particulate personality tests*

This group includes inventories, interest tests, trait rating schemes, diagnostic tests and all such particulate tests that are meant to explore the general qualities, or substantial uniformities, underlying behaviour in any field, but more particularly social behaviour. The addition axiom for this group would be that the sum of n item answers scored for introversion, neuroticism, job adjustment, marital adjustment, mechanical interests, ascendance, and so on, equals the substantial uniformity so defined and that this can be transferred to the appropriate real situations. This group of tests would therefore replace groups 2, 3 and 4 and possibly 5 if its claims could be established. But, following MacIver's discussion [41, Ch. 5] of empiricist rating schemes one can only say that the definition of the substantial uniformity tested is impeccably operational; one cannot go on to specify in what real situations it would be found. If one looks for it, one finds that empirical studies of validity, that would give some indirect evidence with regard to transfer, are not extensive enough to be conclusive; but they tend quite uniformly in the same direction. The review of these methods by Cronbach [15, Chs. 13 and 14], and similar reviews in other texts, mention validities that are quite high enough for various of the methods to be useful in selection, for example, but not nearly high enough to establish more than that the test and the criterion performance have something not very extensive (up to perhaps 30 per cent of their variance) in common. It is known, for example, that persons in different occupational groups are significantly differentiated by interest tests and also by some tests of the inventory type which include items of generalized or abstract social behaviour. But a merely significant, or highly significant, differentiation is not nearly sufficient to warrant the assumption that the differentiating items do represent at all closely the interests of engineers, for example, as contrasted with musicians, or the social habits of salesmen as contrasted with bookkeepers. The assumption, indeed, is unlikely, for both interests and social habits are in real life organized and coherent in a way that bears no obvious resemblance to the forced comparison of badly set out fragments that the test requires.

The same kind of reservation must be made with regard to the validities reported in the other main field in which work has been done, that of diagnostic testing. Here too significant differentiation among kinds of disorder or between maladjusted and normal persons is not sufficient to support the transfer of differentiating items to real behaviour. Even when these items are apparently statements of symptoms a simple transfer is, indeed, hardly to be expected; for the symptoms of a disorder too are organized in a coherent system and are not merely unrelated bits with a uniform weight.

Besides the limited studies of validity, there are other indications that the fragmentation of behaviour makes transfer impossible. The low correlations sometimes reported between different tests that are supposed to measure the same quality may mean only that the operational definition of that quality is sound (i.e. neuroticism is what is measured by this test) but this itself implies that the name given to the quality is almost an arbitrary convention. If the two heaps of items do not even resemble each other in a case in which the test constructors have good logical reasons for expecting them to do so, it is not likely that either heap can resemble real behaviour. Conversely, it can be argued that high correlations between supposedly independent qualities show the failure of fragmentation. Cronbach [15, p. 397] reports a typical case of industrial merit rating in which the twelve qualities rated are quite highly correlated (from 0·25 to 0·88) although the correlations between paired raters are low (from 0·35 to 0·48). This he interprets as showing a large halo effect together with other large errors. An alternative interpretation is that the raters found it impossible to distinguish the twelve supposedly independent qualities but attempted the fragmentation of the single overall judgement of competence that they would naturally make at the cost of their accuracy. This interpretation is supported by the fact that the split half correlation for the whole set of ratings would be 0·90 or more, a figure which could hardly be attained unless the raters were rating substantially the same thing in twelve slightly different disguises.

One may conclude that the addition axiom has been shown to be distinctly improbable in the few special fields where it has been indirectly investigated. It is therefore even less probable in more ordinary and more complex fields. Family behaviour, for example, and even actual behaviour at work are not likely to bear any noticeable resemblance to the items of marital adjustment or job adjustment inventories, despite the strictly operational definition of the qualities that these inventories measure. The addition axiom, indeed, is so unlikely in the light of common experience that one could more reasonably reject it in the absence of positive supporting evidence than wait until it is disproved. In this respect the methods of group 7 are not to be compared with the indirect methods, which have a reasonable promise of transferability (though by analogy, not by addition) even though they have not been sufficiently investigated.

Group 8. *Particulate cognitive tests*

This group includes all tests requiring some kind of fragmentary intellectual behaviour, from the varied crossword puzzles of intelligence tests through the radio quiz items of achievement tests to the items of clerical classification tests. The addition axiom here is that the sum of n items scored for intelligence or some other operationally defined quality equals an examination performance, a job performance or some kind of general competence in handling one's affairs. As this group includes the oldest and best established psychological tests of any kind, studies of validity are abundant and they all show that the addition axiom is improbable. The inadequacy of intelligence test scores as a basis for classifying mental defectives is due to the fact that ignorance of simple words and inability to solve simple puzzles does not necessarily mean that the person cannot manage his affairs. The quite low (though significant and therefore useful) discrimination between occupations that the tests of this group give shows that performance even in widely different occupations (e.g. intellectual as against manual) depends to a not very different degree on the fragmentary recall of synonyms or analysis of diagrams, although the organized and coherent use of these fragments in the two occupational groups is doubtless very different. Lastly, the rather low correlations between particulate cognitive tests and examination criteria at various levels, especially the higher, show that fragmentary intellectual operations do not add to make a connected argument. There are exceptions to this, in cases where the examination performance is itself fragmentary; but the high validities found in these special cases are an example of analogical transfer and not of addition. One could therefore put the special sub-group of analogous aptitude tests into group 3, were it not that the very abstract nature of both test and criterion disqualifies them for this.

It may be concluded that the evidence against the addition axiom in this field is considerable enough for it to be rejected. It follows that the exploration of real intellectual behaviour remains the function of the speculative and largely hypothetical methods of group 6.

Group 9. *Particulate psychophysical tests*

This group includes simple paper apparatus tests of cancellation, dotting and so on, apparatus tests that are meant to analyse or simulate a job for which persons are being selected, and laboratory procedures used for investigating perceptual and motor functions. These tests are particulate in that they require repeated performance on identical or similar items, and the evidence about them is fairly extensive (cf. Cronbach [15, pp. 216–223] and Viteles [70, Chs. 13

and 14]). The simpler repetitive tests of manipulation are fairly valid for jobs requiring repetitive manipulation; in this case there is no question of the addition of fragments as there is only the one operation, and this can apparently be transferred by analogy. Analytic tests of perceptual or motor functions, whether simple laboratory tests (such as perceptual speed or reaction time) or complex specially devised tests (such as multiple co-ordination, aiming tests and so on) are of very low validity for any kind of job. Two perceptions and three consecutive movements add to make only a small part of a real co-ordinated performance. Tests that closely simulate a real job, however, are much more valid so long as the person has enough practice on them to reach a reliable performance; that is, a steady rate of climb, if not a level performance. But if the test (and the job) are complex the person takes so long to do this that he is practically trained to do the actual job before his performance can be measured. In this respect these tests resemble the more valid repetitive tests of manipulation, though the latter, of course, need give the person only a short training, as is required for the job. With the complex work-sample test also, therefore, there is no addition of fragments but only a transfer by close analogy. The tests in group 9 which are capable of analogical transfer would indeed be better placed in group 3, among the enacted situations, if it were not for their limited and highly specialized function. It is on the whole reasonable to regard these tests as having a high degree of substantial abstraction because their counterparts in real life are rare. The case is different with the analytic tests in group 9: for them the addition axiom is clearly even less tenable than it is for cognitive tests.

Conclusion

A general conclusion to the discussion of substantial abstraction may be briefly stated. Economical methods of enquiry must be capable of wide application to areas of real behaviour and must give results that can be transferred to those areas with some confidence. Economy in this sense is achieved only by methods that are work samples in so far as they require the person to enact behaviour analogous to that which is to be investigated. The direct methods of group 2 require him to enact an actual sample of his behaviour when he is observed and to enact real situations in his head, as it were, when he is interviewed. The interview is thus an effective work sample when it is conducted as a controlled but continuously developing drama with a cast of two, according to the rules set out long since by Roethlisberger and Dickson [57, Ch. 13]. Much the same is true of the indirect methods. Those of group 4 back up the interview by getting the person to enact certain kinds of analytic behaviour

131

and those of group 3 require him to act openly in situations that, as Maier [41, Ch. 4] implies, differ from real situations only in being removed from their normal locus. The methods of group 5 require the person to work at expressing his sub-intentional behaviour and those of group 6 to reproduce his articulate intellectual behaviour. The indirect methods too require some personal skill, but only for their introduction, as their development is carried out by the person alone.

That is as far as one can go in substantial abstraction. The abstract methods of groups 7, 8 and 9 are on the whole quicker to construct, use and analyse than are the other methods, especially the direct methods, which are the most tedious. The abstract methods are also easier to use, as no personal skill is necessary beyond that of the clerk who follows the routine down to the last comma. In the simpler aspects of economy, the abstract methods are certainly superior. But they sample nothing beyond the abstract behaviour which they include so that, whatever their practical or applied uses, they are disqualified as methods of enquiry by their very low precision. The place to strike a compromise between convenience and precision is between the indirect and the abstract methods; that is to say, between the methods which are all necessary (for direct methods must be backed up by indirect) and methods that are not clearly even useful.

It may be as well to make it clear that this conclusion applies to the methods of 'experimental psychology'. These methods have not been explicitly mentioned, partly because investigation outside the laboratory is both more common and more important, but chiefly because, as methods, there is nothing special about them. The majority of the methods reviewed by Woodworth and Schlosberg [73], for example, depend on the use of psychophysical apparatus, ranging in complexity from a touch-bristle to a large machine. All of these are ordinary methods of group 9, in the same way as the fragmentary intellectual tasks used in some learning experiments are ordinary methods of group 8. However rigorously controlled the experiments are in which any of these methods are used, they have nothing to do with ordinary behaviour. It is true that there are other 'experimental' methods. The interesting projective techniques of free association, the judgement of facial expression and telling the subject gruesome stories, (Woodworth and Schlosberg [73, Chs. 3, 5 and 6 respectively]) clearly belong in group 5, together with the properly developed projective tests. Similarly, the material to which the 'methods' of scaling, rating, ranking or paired comparisons are applied [73, Ch. 9] could be in groups 4 or 7, depending on its nature. What matters in this case, as in others, is firstly whether an intelligent question has been framed and not merely whether it has been presented under meticulous control.

132

INSTRUMENTAL DEFINITION AND SYNTHETIC ABSTRACTION

THE nature of psychological enquiry has been clarified somewhat by the discussion of substantial abstraction. An efficient enquiry will be directed to whatever areas or parts of areas of ordinary behaviour may be of interest, will use direct methods to investigate intentional behaviour in these areas and will use indirect methods both to assist this investigation and to investigate the sub-intentional and intellectual behaviour that are the ground of behaviour in all areas. Thus far, then, psychology is committed to rather elaborate enquiry, certainly to a more elaborate kind of enquiry than is ever contemplated in the use of the established abstract methods. It may be possible to simplify the procedures outlined by making other abstractions. Instrumental definition, beyond the least degree that is necessary for any particular method, would reduce the variety of material that the method gets. Synthetic abstraction at the first stage, or categorical abstraction in ordering the material, would reduce its variety further, and statistical abstraction in analysing the data, the second state of synthetic abstraction, would make yet a third reduction. Whether or not these reductions together, or any one by itself, would be compatible with efficiency in the enquiry is the question that must be considered; for however common it may be to make further abstractions, the practice cannot be accepted only on the simple ground of convenience.

INSTRUMENTAL DEFINITION AND CATEGORICAL ABSTRACTION

In considering the two procedures that abstract from the variety of the data by using pre-determined classifications, one must note

133

that the first of these, instrumental definition, is to some extent inevitable in the use of any deliberate method of enquiry. Condensed acquaintance is possible only if, in taking a brief section of the vast diversity of behaviour, one directs the person's attention to the kind of answer which is wanted as well as to the area of interest. This is obvious with the indirect methods. Projective tests, for example, are used because one cannot get at the person's ordinary sub-intentional behaviour directly (except perhaps in psychoanalysis); but, in accepting this degree of substantial abstraction, one has also to accept the definition of the person's responses by the instrument used. His test behaviour is not sub-intentional behaviour in all areas or at large, it is sub-intentional behaviour with certain inkblots, pictures, words and so on. The same is true even of the interview. The interviewer does not sit down with the person and wait in silence or say only: 'Talk'. Whatever value these procedures might have as projective tests they would miss the purpose of the interview, which is to get the person talking about things specified by the interviewer. The specification may be vague or precise, but even if it is vague the instrument defines a limited range within which the person can operate. Instrumental definition, however, may be taken deliberately beyond this minimum degree. Four stages may be distinguished in the general case, without reference to any particular kind of method.

1. The experimenter directs the person's attention to what is to be done, but does not observe, or may even deliberately avoid, either a fixed order of work or a fixed form of instructions.
2. Order of work and detailed instructions for work are fixed, but the person invents or constructs the response; that is, he selects it from the whole range available in his knowledge or imagination.
3. As stage 2, with the addition that the person selects each response from a set presented to him by the experimenter, but without reference to other responses.
4. As stage 3, with the addition that the person selects responses to fit a categorical order presented by the experimenter: e.g. he is told to avoid 'doubtful' responses as much as possible or to put not more than a tenth, or not less than a fifth, of his responses in the central category of a scale.

Instrumental definition may be followed by categorical abstraction, which depends on the experimenter's ideas of the best way of reducing the data gathered to some kind of orderly system. In this process, four stages may be distinguished which are similar to those of instrumental definition.

1. The experimenter classifies the data by the natural differences and resemblances found in a content analysis and without reference to any one system of variables or set of dimensions. This stage (examples of which are given in the following discussion) does involve abstraction because it is necessary, at the least, to decide which differences are important and which are not.
2. The classification of data is referred to a set of variables which is selected without reference to the data, on general or theoretical grounds, and which specifies qualities but not categories of these qualities. For example, the scheme requires that the data be referred to the needs of nurturance and abasement, but leaves it to be determined by analysis how these shall be rated; so that heaped or U-shaped symmetrical distributions, or asymmetrical or even two-dimensional distributions are equally permissible so long as they represent the data efficiently.
3. The variables and categories are fixed before analysis. In this stage it is laid down that the need of nurturance will be rated as high, low or absent, or as very high, high, and low or absent, whatever shape distributions these rating schemes produce. In stage 2, either of these schemes would do and the choice between them would depend on which gave the best representation of the data for the purpose of the analysis.
4. The variables, categories and distributions are fixed before analysis. It is decided that job attitudes, as they appear in the interview or questionnaire record, will be rated on a five point scale with equal sub-frequencies, so that the most favourable fifth of all the attitudes expressed are put in the top category, whatever that may be called: and so on.

Categorical abstraction could therefore be called instrumental definition after the event, but the processes are distinguished on practical grounds. They are successive, rather than independent processes, for an advanced stage of instrumental definition can only be followed by an equally advanced stage of categorical abstraction, whereas the first stage of definition may be followed by any stage of abstraction. A mental test with multiple choice answers, for example (stage 3 of definition), is almost necessarily at stage 3 of abstraction; for the items are the variables and the right and wrong answers are the categories. Even in this case, however, the experimenter has some freedom of action because he can analyse the actual answers selected in conjunction with a criterion, making no decision on which answers belong in the good and bad categories till he has investigated this. He then operates at stage 2 of abstraction. With the least defined methods, of course, there is no determined passage to abstraction;

the open interview, for example, can be analysed at any stage of abstraction. The fact that abstraction follows on from definition, but not uniformly, gives the practical ground for regarding these as two distinct processes instead of eight elements of one process. Instrumental definition decides what the person will do and is final and irretrievable; if it makes a method of enquiry inefficient, analysis cannot improve the situation even where it is to some extent possible to avoid categorical abstraction. The latter process, however, only decides what the person has done and is therefore always retrievable if it is applied by itself; if the analysis appears to be useless it can always be re-worked. That is why this process is logically classed as the first stage of synthetic abstraction.

However, if the practical distinction is important in the construction or selection of particular methods of enquiry, the two processes are conveniently taken together in discussing their general bearing on methods, both because they have similar effects and because they are usually applied together. In the following account, the various possible combinations of instrumental definition and categorical abstraction are taken in relation to each of the main methods of enquiry in turn. For shortness, the combinations are referred to by numbers without titles: thus (1, 1) means the combination of stage 1 of instrumental definition with stage 1 of categorical abstraction, and so on.

Instrumental definition	*Categorical abstraction*			
	1. Open content-analysis	2. Only variables fixed before analysis	3. Variables and categories fixed	4. Variables categories and distributions fixed
1. Order of work and responses open	2, 3, 4,			
2. Task defined, responses open	2, 3, 4, 5, 6,			
3. Task defined, forced choice responses	4	7, 9	4, 8, 9	
4. Task, responses and distribution defined				

136

The preceding table may be of use in clarifying the argument. In this, the rows are the four stages of instrumental definition and the columns the four stages of categorical abstraction. The number entries in the table are the groups of methods, as described in Chapter 9, and these are placed where they properly fall according to the following discussion, but other possible placings are not shown. For example, in the second row of the first column the number 5 is entered (among others) and is entered nowhere else. This means that the methods of group 5 are regarded as being properly at stage 2 of instrumental definition and stage 1 of categorical abstraction: and that any other placing is undesirable.

Group 2. Interviewing and observation. These direct methods fall naturally at (1, 1), though the exigencies of recording may take them to (1, 2). The recording even of an interview is necessarily selective, if it flows at all and unless a machine is used; and the recorder must to some extent select in accordance with his preconceived and possibly unanalysed ideas of the importance or unimportance of various kinds of remark, although he may be able to select mostly by recording only the bare skeleton of what the person says. The interview may be at (2, 1), in part only, if it has been found that some questions are best asked in exactly the same words for all persons. The general questions about social classes that were used by Oeser and Hammond [50, Ch. 20] are an example: opinions of this kind may be distorted by variations in the wording. The interview may be further abstracted by instrumental definition for the sake of economy in working. The interview which uses a fixed schedule throughout (like some employment interviews) is at (2, 1) and so are open-answer questionnaires that refer to real behaviour in a systematically presented context (like the 'Day at home' questionnaire used by Oeser and Hammond [50, Ch. 9] and Oeser and Emery [51, Ch. 7]). The questionnaire can easily be taken to (3, 3) or possibly (3, 2): and (3, 4) and (4, 4) are unlikely but logically similar variants of this.

These economies are doubtful. Except for the fixed schedule interview, all the methods mentioned are considerably faster than others in group 2, as they can be used with large numbers of persons at the same time and all therefore probably gain about equally in speed, though the questionnaire at (2, 1) may be slowed down somewhat by the answers being open. It is the precision of these methods which is doubtful. All are bound to lose some information, as the experimenter cannot explore the person's behaviour with further questions and the person is, at the least, prevented from following what may be his natural course. This is true even of the fixed schedule interview at (2, 1), which has no considerable advantage in speed anyway. The only possible case for this method is that it cuts down variations between incompetent or relatively untrained interviewers. However, such persons need not be employed, and even if they are it seems doubtful whether the removal of irrelevant differences, at the cost of removing relevant ones between the persons interviewed by reducing the variety of the material, is really a gain. The loss of variety, of course, is much greater with the questionnaire at (3, 3), or its equivalents. With these, variety is positively excluded by the structure of the method and, as MacIver [41, p. 208] observes, the material is of very doubtful use for the inference of intentional perceptions. Equally, the transferability of findings is much reduced. The only conceivable way to avoid the reduction of variety in the material would be to construct questionnaires in which every possible aspect of the real behaviour being studied was described and every possible alternative response was stated. It need hardly be said that this procedure is not proposed seriously. Besides that it would break up the connectedness of the person's behaviour and probably bore him excessively, it would be so laborious in the stage of construction that it might waste, rather than gain, time.

It may be concluded that, while there is no case for the use of the fixed schedule interview, the questionnaire at (2, 1) is a reasonable compromise, in special circumstances and for limited areas of real behaviour only, between speed and precision. Any of the more defined methods may be chosen if speed is the chief consideration, almost regardless of precision; but one must be clear that this is the only possible ground for using them. Their instrumental definition (and consequent categorical abstraction) make them of little more use, even when they are directed to coherent and defined areas of behaviour, than the methods of group 7, in which areas of behaviour are confounded in a miscellaneous sample. It is indeed not unlikely that the more defined methods discussed would be better classed in group 7.

The next point to consider is categorical abstraction, so far as it is not involved in definition; that is, as applied to undefined material, especially to the open interview. In case (1, 2) the interview records are reduced to a set of variables arranged at the beginning of work. If this is taken beyond the abstraction which is involved in recording, information may be lost. It is decided, for example, that 'attitude to job' will include remarks made by a number of workers interviewed about any aspect of the job itself; how they like it generally, what they like or dislike about it, what they think of the physical conditions of work, any suggestions they make for alterations in work processes and anything else that might be classified under the same head. Remarks may be made about several of these topics and the decision that the one variable must include them all compels the choice between two awkward ways of handling the data. The variable may be treated as compound or multi-dimensional, including such categories as 'likes the job itself but not the physical conditions' and 'dislikes the job, does/does not suggest alterations'. Compound variables of this kind are quite acceptable in principle. Especially with interview material, a judicious use of compound variables may well be necessary in order to represent the connectedness of the person's reported behaviour or opinions. But compounding cannot be taken beyond the limit of convenience. A variable that included remarks on so many topics (even if some were rarely mentioned) would probably have an unmanageably large number of uninterpretably complex categories. Information would be lost by the blurring of the relations between the distinguishable aspects of satisfaction with the actual job. The alternative is that the blurring could be done directly by rating all remarks, of whatever kind and in whatever combination, on a one-dimensional scale. The loss of information in this case is obvious.

The other important case is (1, 3), an example of which would be the use of the one variable, 'relations with fellow workers', with the three categories good, neutral and bad, to include all remarks on how the workers interviewed get on with their fellow workers and on how much they have to do with them. It may be found that many workers fit easily into the three categories provided. But there are some who particularly state that, while they are on good terms with their fellow workers they have little to do with them from choice (avoid common social activities, take care to have no particular friends and so on). These persons fit neither into the 'good' nor into the 'neutral' category. They just cannot be included unless the case is pushed back to (1, 2) and the variable made into a compound by adding a new category of 'good but on distant terms'. But even if this is done, there is still no provision for the foreign workers interviewed, most of whom state that they have nothing to do with their fellow workers because they cannot speak English. The one Greek in a small section may be striving hard to establish contact with his mates, using his less than basic English; or he may be suspicious of them and keep his distance or simply indifferent to his isolation. He could be classified under any of these three heads, but he cannot be fitted into any of the categories even of the compound variable.

It may be concluded that categorical abstraction by itself involves some loss of information for a doubtful gain, if any gain, in speed of working the analysis. This is not a serious consideration, however, with interview material; serious and sustained mistakes about the best set of variables to use are unlikely, as the variables are probably apparent in an inspection of the records. Even the two cases taken are unlikely, and case (1, 4) is so unlikely that it need not be considered. The mixed cases (2, 2), (2, 3) and (2, 4) might occur but need not be discussed as with them little more can be lost than is lost in the stage of instrumental definition.

The other group 2 method, observation, requires only a brief note. It is usual to manage the complexity of observable behaviour by sampling it and by recording only specifiable and countable aspects of behaviour (cf. Cronbach, [15, pp. 390, 393]). These procedures may be regarded as stages 2 and 3 respectively of instrumental definition, for in this case the experimenter's order of work and the set of responses he can choose from are fixed in the same way as these are fixed for the person being interviewed. The remarks made about interviewing therefore apply equally to observation, if not more strongly, as the very purpose of scientific procedures in this case is to break up by selection the connectedness of actual and not merely of reported behaviour.

Group 3. The staged situation. This falls naturally at (1, 1) or at (2, 1) depending on how detailed the instructions are. Recording is necessarily selective to some extent and this tends to take the method to (3, 1). This move is clearly made, however, only if recording is deliberately selective on a pre-arranged scheme. In this case the enacted situation is observed in much the same way as in ordinary behaviour, in that the experimenter's instrument defines what he can see. In this case also categorical abstraction is almost certain to be involved for, if only some actions or remarks (e.g. those denoting hostility, persuasiveness, tact and so on) are recorded, there is that much less content to analyse and the case is probably at (3, 2) to (3, 4). Where selective recording is used in order to make a general rating of the person's adequacy (as a foreman, potential executive, etc.) the case is clearly at (3, 3) or (3, 4). Deliberately selective recording thus has the same effect as the categorical abstraction of a full record (case (1, 3) or (2, 3)), though this is retrievable.

There is no obvious case for these abstractions. With the staged situation, speed of work is hardly a point, as it is staged in order to save the time that would be necessary to observe ordinary behaviour. In any case, recording can be accelerated only by accelerating the action. The most selective recording is no faster than the least selective and the abstract analysis of records is no faster than is a treatment depending on a careful content analysis. The loss of information by abstraction is likely to be serious. The inference of intentional perceptions in the staged situation and especially the transfer of these to real life situations depend critically on the situation's closely resembling a real life situation; only if it does can it be accepted as a group 3 method of enquiry. There is not much point in arranging a good imitation of real life if the record of the imitation is reduced to a bald summary of general qualities that could be inferred no more doubtfully by using an abstract method.

Group 4. The hypothetical situation. The effect of the two processes under consideration on the methods of this group is much the same as their effect on the interview, as these methods are extensions of the interview. Certain differences among the particular methods reviewed in Chapter 9 may be noted.

The most open of these are the question about things that might be changed in a factory, the hypothetical diagnostic question and the question about the best and worst things that could happen (which are (c), (d) and (e) respectively in Chapter 9). These fall naturally at (1, 1) or at (2, 1) if they require specific wording. As their effectiveness depends on their being open, instrumental definition would simply turn them into items in an abstract questionnaire. Categorical abstraction alone is less serious, as it is no more likely to be applied in this case than it is to the ordinary interview.

Two other examples of this group, the questionnaire about good and bad things to do at home and the question about a man's main aims in life (which are (a) and (b) respectively in Chapter 9) are more defined. Their effectiveness, as presented by Oeser and Hammond [50, Chs. 14 and 18] and Oeser and Emery [51, Ch. 8], depends on the careful choice of their wording, so that their natural position is at (2, 1). These methods too, however, are probably reduced in efficiency by any further instrumental definition. In this case, again, categorical abstraction alone need hardly be considered.

The remaining two methods are the hypothetical question in the opinion poll and the paired comparisons of a number of jobs ((f) and (g), respectively, in Chapter 9). These are the most defined methods of group 4. The opinion poll is at (3, 1) or (3, 3), depending on the kind of question asked, and the paired comparisons schedule is at (3, 3). The question of further instrumental definition or categorical abstraction therefore hardly arises, but the contrast between the two methods is interesting. The paired comparisons schedule is at (3, 3) because this is necessary in order to force the person to make a critical evaluation of the whole range of jobs presented. Used in conjunction with other methods, this is a sound group 4 method. The opinion poll question, however, is at or beyond (3, 1) merely because asking it in this form is quicker. If the question is remotely hypothetical, it may be doubted whether the answers are as meaningful as those that would be got in an open interview. This procedure may well belong rather to group 7 because of its over-definition.

It may be concluded that the methods of group 4 are no more

likely to be reduced in efficiency by instrumental definition or categorical abstraction than are those of group 2. These processes, however, do impair efficiency if taken beyond the necessary minimum and their general effect is to reduce the methods considered to forms more appropriately placed in group 7.

Group 5. Contextless projective tests. These methods must be at stage 2 of instrumental definition, for they are test methods with defined instructions and procedures. Definition beyond this stage, however, is never proposed, for it is obvious that including multiple choice responses would disqualify these tests as projective tests and would place them in group 7 or possibly in group 8. Their natural position, therefore, is at (2, 1) but the categorical abstraction of their results in the usual scoring procedures takes them to (2, 3) or (2, 4).

The Thematic Apperception Test, for example, may be scored by rating traits that the person is supposed to have projected into his stories or by classifying the characters of the stories, and identifying and perhaps rating needs, presses and so on. Both these procedures use preconceived schemes of analysis, for the general classification of characters and general schemes of needs and presses are not necessarily more applicable to a particular set of records than is the simpler trait-rating scheme. The Rorschach Test is handled somewhat differently. The scoring proper depends on the original content analysis, as revised by Rorschach's successors, and this was evidently an empirical analysis. The interpretation of the scored record, however, proceeds through the use of rather vague and inefficient statistical indices to an overall impressionistic description of personality. The test as used is thus removed from (2, 1) to (2, 3).

It is notorious that for both these tests there is little agreement between scorers who use the procedures outlined, so that the results, as Cronbach [15, pp. 448, 449] observes, are hardly capable of serious testing in relation to other information and have shown no relations of any importance. But agreement on the scoring of Rorschach records taken by itself (that is, only on the classification of responses) is reasonably close and the empirical validity of the 'neurotic signs', which are items derived from the scored record statistically and not by interpretation, in relation to other diagnoses has been found to be reasonably high in some cases. This suggests that the usefulness of these tests has been obscured by scoring procedures which, however suitable they may be for clinical diagnosis, are not suitable for the purpose of general investigation. At all events, it is possible that a detailed item-validation of the Rorschach Test against a range of other information (or criteria) would clarify its working and perhaps improve the content analysis. With the Thematic Apperception

Test, clarification would require a careful empirical content analysis, followed by item validation.

Projective tests are important enough to warrant a demonstration of the possibilities of content analysis by reference to the test material discussed in Chapter 9 in relation to the transferability of findings. Here the point to demonstrate is how the content analysis is done, and for this purpose four examples of stories about the Thematic Apperception Test picture 6BM (Mother and Son) may be taken first.

(i) The son leaves to make his way in the world, all ends well. 'The boy has just been paid off, and is worried how to break the news to his mother. He finally tells her, however, to find that she understands perfectly and makes him feel good. He promptly goes round the agencies to find work and lands a job as a salesman. In a short time he discovers his bent is salesmanship and in a year's time he is a branch manager for his firm. Now he is head of a large sales organization and all new salesmen are given a thorough training by him.'

(ii) The son is a bad lot, all ends well. 'Jack went out for the evening, and met some old friends, drink followed drink, and he finished up in the police cells; on being released he went home and confessed to his mother, she was disgusted and from this, so was he, and self-disgust turned him to decency.'

(iii) The son is thinking of getting married, no conclusion. 'Frank has arrived home with the news that he is going to marry Joan. His mother who loves him very much is very upset because she believes Joan to be unworthy of her son. Frank cannot accept this view but is very grieved that he should hurt his mother and is puzzled as to how he can still marry Joan and yet not upset his mother. He is . . .' (unfinished).

(iv) Family drama, ends miserably. 'The young man, happily married, has just returned from the hospital. His wife, having just had a baby, has just died in giving birth to it, and bewildered, he returns to his mother full of grief and not quite able to understand why this sort of thing should be allowed to happen. His mother knows just how he feels, and just cannot say anything with which to console him.'

These examples show the four themes and three outcomes that were used to classify a sample of 100 stories. The only assumption required by the content analysis is that there is a detectable order of natural differences among the stories, so that each resembles some others more in both its theme and its outcome than it resembles the

143

remainder. The analysis is therefore at stage 1 of categorical abstraction, for it is not decided in advance that theme and outcome will be the variables, or compound variable, used (as it would be in stage 2), nor that the categories of these variables will be as described (stage 3), nor that the frequencies in categories will have a specified distribution (stage 4). The same points may be demonstrated by reference to the briefer material of the word-association test, taken from the same source. The classification of responses to the word 'beer', first in a list of fifty, has seven categories with titles, examples and frequencies as set out below.

1. Social uses. 'Music and lounge'   21
2. Personal reference: definitely accepted. 'I like beer'   11
3.   ,,   ,,   : vaguely accepted. 'Drink for health'   19
4.   ,,   ,,   : accepted but criticized. 'Poor quality now'   8
5.   ,,   ,,   : qualified acceptance. 'Jolly good in moderation' 8
6.   ,,   ,,   : rejected. 'Beer is best—left alone'   12
7. Expository words and phrases. 'Bar'   21

The least necessary assumption of a natural order of differences and resemblances was of course made in this case too. Thus 'evenings off on a course' was put in category 1, not 2, although it includes the latter: and 'over rated by many' was put in category 6 although it could possibly refer to 5.

The content analysis of 100 cases by one experimenter does not show, of course, whether the schemes arrived at for either test would be applicable to larger samples or whether they could be conveniently communicated to other experimenters. However, if one person can do what Sheldon [60, p. 36] in another context calls 'getting some good intuitions', presumably others can too. The point is that the analysis of these tests by conventional trait-rating methods was tried and the results were unrelated to any other data from the selection procedure in which the tests were used, while the results of the analysis outlined above were reasonably related to other data. Two findings may be added to those mentioned in Chapter 9. In the selection procedure, the psychologists and the service testing officers (as well as other board members), made overall judgements of the person's officer potential. The psychologists' judgements depended partly on the impressionistic analysis of the projective tests but on much more besides this, and the testing officers' judgements were made without reference to this material at all; and the two judgements are only moderately correlated. It is found that a scale derived from the analysis of responses to one picture and five words is fifty per cent better than chance at predicting the psychologists' judgements in the three categories acceptable, possible and unacceptable.

An equivalent (not identical) scale is seventy-two per cent better than chance in predicting the testing officers' judgements. These are findings for a test of six items, that would take six minutes or so to administer if they could be given by themselves. It is clear that this test, and therefore much more so the whole tests, did elicit responses that were related to persistent and important elements in the person's behaviour; but the relation is found only if categorical abstraction is taken no further than stage 1. With further abstraction, the information is simply lost.

It may be concluded that, as the usual objections to the projective tests of group 5 may be valid only if abstract methods of analysis are used, it is an unfortunate accident of history that these methods are so common. It seems unlikely that they are even faster than is an empirical content analysis or than a scoring scheme would be that was based on such an analysis.

Group 6. Projective tests with a fantasy context. The methods placed in this group because they are too fantastic to be in group 3 hardly require comment. Instrumental definition and categorical abstraction would have the same effect on them as on the method of group 3, but substantial abstraction has the greater effect in reducing their usefulness.

Groups 7 to 9. Particulate tests generally. These groups may be taken together in order to point out certain contrasts with the other groups or methods. All the methods in these groups are substantially abstracted to a high degree, for the sake of speed in working as well as on theoretical grounds; and all are abstracted in other respects for the same reasons, especially the former. The particulate personality tests of group 7 fall naturally at $(3, 2)$ but may be at $(3, 3)$ if logical instead of empirical scoring is used. The particular cognitive tests of group 8 are usually at $(3, 3)$, rarely at $(2, 3)$, when the answers are invented, not selected, and even more rarely at $(3, 2)$, when the items are empirically validated. The particulate psychophysical tests of group 9 are at $(3, 2)$ or $(3, 3)$, depending on how one defines a variable and a category, but regardless of the fact that the response is in a sense created, for the very narrow range of variation possible in most such tests is not enough to place them at $(2, 2)$ or $(2, 3)$.

In all these cases, further instrumental definition or categorical abstraction would make little or no difference if they could be done at all. The question, by contrast with other groups of methods, is whether less definition and abstraction, so far as they might be possible, would make the particulate tests more efficient. This seems unlikely. The appropriate case would be the personality questionnaire or intelligence test at $(2, 1)$: that is, with invented answers followed by an empirical content analysis and empirical validation. Such tests would take longer to establish, though no longer to score once they were established, than the usual more abstracted forms. They would be more efficient only if it were easier to infer real intentional or real intellectual behaviour, in the respective cases, from the results. The substantial abstraction of these tests makes this inference so unlikely that less abstraction in handling the results could hardly retrieve the position. A miscellaneous heap of quiz answers or of fragmentary facts and memories could hardly be turned into connected behaviour merely by the more careful sorting of the bits.

It may be concluded generally that neither instrumental definition nor categorical abstraction is important with the less efficient, substantially abstract, methods of enquiry. Both processes, however, may impair the usefulness of the less abstract, direct and indirect, methods in so far as they reduce the possibility of inferring intentional behaviour or of transferring findings to real situations. In this sense these processes reduce efficiency and they do so for the sake of no marked gain in speed or no gain at all.

Instrumental definition is perhaps the less objectionable process, as it is not often taken beyond the least stage which is necessary for a method to work at all. Definition beyond this stage moves the method down in the order of substantial abstraction into the groups of abstract methods. But this process necessarily involves the more advanced stages of categorical abstraction also, and this process is the more objectionable in that it may be inappropriately applied by itself and give a poor treatment of good material. This is not likely to be done with interview material (of groups 2 or 4) unless the interview is a schedule with a check list for ratings, which is merely a group 7 questionnaire administered individually, so that categorical abstraction at stage 3 is involved anyway. This process may be overdone in observing behaviour (groups 2 and 3) and has been overdone, with unfortunate effects, with contextless projective tests (group 5). Its general effect is to confound the natural order of the data by fitting them into a classification that is likely to be really suitable only by chance and may be grossly unsuitable.

STATISTICAL ABSTRACTION

The next matter to consider is the effect on the various methods of enquiry of the statistical treatment of their results. It could be said that categorical abstraction is the necessary preliminary to statistical treatment, for it is the first or second step in reducing chaos

146

to order and the final step is measurement, or the inference of mathematical relations. This final step, which is called statistical abstraction, does depend on categorical abstraction, which is why the two processes are classed together logically as elements in synthetic abstraction. In the particular kind of statistical analysis which is called abstract, the assumptions that the variable categories have continuous order and specifiable intervals (which are made in categorical abstraction) are followed by the third assumption that the variables denote additive qualities.

However, if this is the most common kind of statistical analysis, it is only one kind. Another possibility is that only additive qualities, and not continuous order or specifiable intervals, are assumed for the variables to be analysed, though the two latter assumptions must be made for the final summed variables. The third possibility is that not even additive qualities are assumed. Statistical analysis is used only as MacIver [41, Ch. 14] describes it, to clear the ground for the causal analysis of intentions, and variables are not added.

The choice among these methods of statistical analysis depends on what kind of psychological laws one hopes or expects to be able to derive, and especially on one's preference for causal (intentional) laws or for the more common abstract mathematical laws. It is important to note here that the latter laws, which might be better called quasi-physical, are mathematical only by analogy. The treatment of behaviour as if it were an object or process with physical dimensions may or may not be useful, but it is a strictly analogical treatment. Behaviour cannot be said to have dimensions merely because the person who has mass behaves in space and time. Apart from the trivial use of the measurement of gross mass (or force), length and time in some psychophysical tests, the only behaviour that has physical dimensions is behaviour regarded from the external point of view of the cerebral physiologist. For all behaviour which concerns psychology (that is, all directly known behaviour), dimensions are only a physical analogy. It hardly matters that this, strictly considered, removes the very foundations of parametric statistical analysis. The logical validity of this analysis is sufficiently tested by its results, and it is clear that psychological measures do, for the most part, behave as if they were physical measures. It is the wider implications of the very idea of measurement that matter, and these cannot be accepted without examination unless the general analogy on which they depend is evidently close.

Closeness is not evident in the three particular analogical assumptions on which measurement depends. Continuous order is perhaps the most acceptable, as the idea of a scale of degrees is widely used outside the sphere of physical measurement. By itself, it asserts only a continuous progression of quantity or intensity in one quality, and can be accepted as a rather loose analogy, in that it cannot apply to cases with overlapping classes (compound variables, as argued above). Even this assumption, then, may sometimes break up the orderly variety of common experience. The second assumption, that intervals between variable categories can be specified (usually, that they are equal) may also be acceptable as a loose analogy. It seems reasonable in most cases to say that there appear to be no marked differences among intervals or in rare cases that there are marked differences. However, these are rather vague statements of analogy only (A is to B as B is to C: or A is to B as B is to E: and so on). To pin them down to the precision of measurement may put a strain on common experience in this case too. On the other hand, once continuous order is assumed, the continuous numbering of categories is probably no more than a conventional device for facilitating arithmetic.

The third assumption, that the variables have additive qualities, is more doubtful; but one must be clear that the doubt is not on merely statistical grounds. The popular statistical methods of correlation, multiple regression, factor analysis and the analysis of variance all require that variables should be reduced to quasi-physical measures that can be added, subtracted, multiplied and divided and that, for simplicity in computing, have a normal distribution for preference. Judging by the enormous technical literature on the subject, one can assume that any variable can be turned into a normally distributed measuring scale, with the aid of a few assumptions and some arithmetic. The technical difficulties of addition, as the basic arithmetical process, may be set aside. It is the psychological validity of the process that is doubtful. Addition depends on the assumption that the things to be added (with equal or unequal weight) are functionally equivalent. There are no logical connections or dependencies among them, only indifferently reversible statistical relations, so that the whole must equal the sum of its parts. Variables such as a number of different attitudes to the major areas in a work field, or to the different members of the person's family who were concerned with his upbringing, can be added to make one inclusive measure such as general attitude to work or general identification with the family of origin. The addition is always possible, of course, but it cannot give the same answer. Two persons with the same score on attitude to work may not have a single identical component score, and lesser differences are bound to be common. Of course one can say that such differences in the pattern or composition of attitudes do not matter and, for various purposes, they may not matter. The point is that they are differences, and that they are suppressed by addition, so that the statements (not added and added) are not and cannot be identical even if they are sometimes equivalent. To say that the whole may be regarded as the sum of its parts is not the same as saying that it is the sum of its parts. This is not a remarkable conclusion, for addition depends on a rather remote analogy. Whether it is simply arithmetical or is done through regression weights or factorial weights, it depends on an analogy with mechanics in the simple addition of lengths or in the resolution of forces in an n-dimensional hyperspace. Both analogies seem rather to belong to the more esoteric regions of experience.

The further consideration of the implications of the idea of measurement must be deferred to Chapter 12. It is sufficient to conclude that there is no reason in its analogical basis for regarding measurement as the method of statistical analysis *par excellence*. It is merely a method, and is to be judged, together with other methods, by its results. The results to be considered here are those that are typical of the different methods of analysis with different kinds of data.

The analysis of *ordered data* may be considered first. The methods of group 2 are like those of their less defined extensions in group 4 and perhaps like those of group 3 in that they produce data in which the variables are obviously not all of the same importance. It is to be assumed, for example, that the main job in a person's life is a more important recurrent fact than where he spends his summer holiday and that how he regards his parents is a more important perception than his opinion of casual childhood acquaintances. Of course some parts of a collection of ordered data may be regarded as functionally equivalent, especially if they are, in effect, responses to the same question repeated in slightly different forms. Thus the person's opinions of the atmosphere, temperature, colour of walls, lighting and floor surface of his place of work need hardly be discriminated unless one stands out sharply as a sore point. The same is obviously true for defined responses such as paired comparisons or responses to an attitude questionnaire with highly correlated (closely similar) items: but these defined group 4 methods are better considered together with other unordered data.

If the data have not been subjected to categorical abstraction, a conservative statistical analysis is possible. This includes only the testing of particular hypotheses about single variables as they stand. The hypotheses may be external to the data (that a certain distribution is drawn from a specified parent distribution) or internal (that certain variables are or are not associated), but in neither case is categorical abstraction carried out. The variables are not reduced to quasi-physical measures and are therefore not added. They are taken

149

as they stand, with complex categories of several dimensions if this is the result of the previous analysis, and tested one by one in the logical dissection of the evidence. This kind of analysis, of course, uses only non-parametric methods, mostly chi-square. It is not possible to give a detailed general description of the method of analysis, for it is more like detective work in the following of particular clues through particular material than it is like a uniform routine of scientific analysis. Many examples of the method are presented by Oeser and Hammond [50] and Oeser and Emery [51], and most of these examples demonstrate the main consequence of the method: that the generalizations (or law-like propositions) it arrives at are intentional or causal analyses presented in words.

It has already been argued that categorical abstraction confounds the natural order of data bearing on real behaviour. Addition, which may be unobjectionable with the less ordered parts of such data, merely completes the confusion by aggregating small indiscriminate heaps into larger ones from which the causal inference of intentions is even less possible. Abstract analysis is hardly in keeping with the apparent purpose of the methods of group 2 (and those taken together with this group) and indeed is therefore hardly likely to be applied to such data. If it were, it would merely take the last step in reducing these methods to those of group 7. Whether or not this should be done depends on the status of the different kinds of psychological law, which is not now in question. It may be noted, finally, that abstract analysis is no faster than conservative analysis.

The statistical treatment of *unordered indirect data* may now be considered. The data derived from the methods of groups 5 and 6, together with the more defined parts of group 4 and possibly group 3, are unordered in that no variable can take logical precedence of another. It is not possible to say that the responses to one inkblot, picture or word, or one comparison between two jobs, are more or less important than any other response or comparison. In this case addition is reasonable and indeed necessary, so that a conservative statistical treatment is impossible. But it has already been argued that categorical abstraction confounds the results at least of the methods of groups 5 and 6. Some categorical abstraction must precede an abstract (or parametric or quasi-physical) analysis, but there are important differences in statistical procedure, depending on when and how the categorical abstraction is done.

Unordered data are usually analysed by reference to a criterion, which can be any kind of valid information (whether parametric or not) which is external to the data. If this is done, two slightly different statistical routines are possible. The more conservative routine uses variables with categories that are assumed only to be distinct in kind and not in continuous order, or with specifiable intervals. These variables are compared with the criterion by means of chi-square (or the t-test, if the criterion is quasi-physical). It is an additive, or parametric, routine in which the addition is deferred to the second stage. The more abstract routine compares scaled variables with the criterion by the use of superior statistics such as product moment or multiserial correlations and the analysis of variance. In the conservative routine, particular categories that are found to be related to job success, popularity in school, neurotic maladjustment and so on, are added by unweighted scoring (these categories score 1, all others score 0) to form a scale. In the abstract routine the scale scores on the variables found to be so related are added, unweighted or more probably by regression weights.

These two statistical procedures give by no means the same results although both finish in mathematical or quasi-physical relations. The statistical procedure itself may import minor differences between the two kinds of result. In so far as it may be possible to relate the results of tests in groups 5 and 6, by inspection, to generalized sub-intentional or intellectual behaviour, this will be easier if the components of the total test score are exactly known. Where specified categories have been added, the components are exactly known but with the addition of whole variables, especially through regression weights, the composition of the whole is less certain.

However, this would be a minor difference. With these methods of enquiry too it is not the addition but the preparation for addition that makes the difference. The addition of categories that have been left in their natural order leads to a mathematical relation from which inferences about behaviour in real situations may be drawn. The addition of categories that have already been confounded by abstraction leads to a mathematical relation which is probably of less precision and from which inferences can hardly be drawn. With unordered data the additive analogy with mechanics must be relied on, but the results of analysis depend on whether it is applied as late and cautiously as possible or as early as possible, in the interest of getting fully quasi-physical relations. It may be added that the more conservative statistical analysis is perhaps the faster, as it uses simpler statistics.

The statistical treatment of *unordered abstract data*, from the methods of groups 7, 8 and 9, needs only brief consideration as an abstract treatment is the only real possibility. Some questionnaire or inventory material in group 7 is empirically validated against a criterion and this could be called a conservative treatment where the scoring categories are determined by this analysis, which is the usual case. In group 8, if the items are validated against a criterion, this is usually done only to determine if the answers already defined as right or wrong (that is, categorically abstracted) are valid for the particular criterion. It is doubtful that a full empirical validation would add anything in this case, and the question does not arise with the methods of group 9, in the nature of their items. It may be concluded that with these groups of methods statistical abstraction as a last process is reasonable and legitimate. The physical analogies of continuous order, specifiable intervals and additive qualities may be not unreasonably applied to indiscriminate heaps of fragmentary behaviour. It is not the gathering of these into conveniently larger heaps that matters, for mathematical laws are the only possibility in this case. This possibility is determined, not by the categorical abstraction that precedes analysis, nor by instrumental definition before that, but by substantial abstraction at the beginning of the enquiry. Once that is done, the question of what kind of law can be derived from the enquiry is closed.

CONCLUSIONS

In conclusion, it may be noted that all three of the processes of abstraction discussed in this chapter depend on the size or scope of the investigation, in that any of them may be more reasonably applied to material drawn from only a small area of behaviour than to material with a wide range. Subject only to this reservation, it can be said that the general effect of all three abstractions is to reduce the direct or indirect methods to abstract methods. In this, their effect is the same as that of substantial abstraction and it may be successive, as a direct or indirect method of enquiry can be reduced in substance equally by instrumental definition or, if this is not done, by synthetic abstraction (categorical and statistical, which go together) after the event. In practice, of course, the decision is usually made at the beginning of the enquiry. If abstractions are used only where they are really useful or necessary, as aids to causal analysis, it may be supposed that the enquiry was intended to lead to a causal analysis. Conversely, if abstractions are fully used throughout, it can be assumed that the aim of the enquiry was to derive mathematical laws from a scientifically designed experiment. The mixed case of an enquiry that begins without major abstractions and then introduces them (e.g. the synthetic abstraction of material from undefined instruments in the direct and indirect groups) may be disregarded, as it is not likely to happen unless the experimenter loses his nerve. The distinction between the two main cases is not that either kind of law, and therefore either of the main methods, conservative and abstract, is clearly superior or more relevant to the purposes of psychology. This question remains to be argued. It is clear, however, that the conservative general routine of enquiry is quite workable and that it makes a fuller use of the data of the direct and indirect methods. It therefore cannot be considered merely as a practical alternative to the quasi-physical scientific procedure which has long been established as the procedure of psychology. The conservative procedure is not another approach, which may or may not be used on practical grounds, including convenience. It is a technically sound approach which gives results very different from those of the conventional procedure: and the decision between the two general procedures, if it must be made, must be made by a consideration of their results.

THE EXTENSION OF THE
EVIDENCE

THE discussion so far of the nature and methods of psychological enquiry suggests that the fundamental question is the nature and scope of psychology, for the respective merits or functions of causal and abstract laws cannot be decided merely on technical grounds. However, the derivation of these laws by different treatments of or different preconceptions about the same evidence is now clear, and the way should be open to discuss the different interpretations of that evidence. This is not so. The discussion of methods of getting and handling evidence has been, implicitly and in places explicitly, referred to certain kinds of evidence only. The discussion at least implies that psychological enquiry is concerned with the person's recurrent behaviour in present situations, as studied by an experimenter. This is so, but it may not be sufficient. Conclusions about the nature of enquiry and the methods of enquiry and therefore about the nature of psychological laws may be different if other kinds of evidence are considered too. It is therefore proposed to consider in turn evidence about the person's history and about his non-recurrent behaviour and evidence as handled by different experimenters.

THE INVESTIGATION OF HISTORY

It may be assumed without argument that the investigation of history is necessary if one wishes to study development and the laws of development. How history should or can be studied for this purpose is a question that may be set aside meantime. The only method that must be excluded is the simultaneous study of groups of persons of different ages. This kind of study is quite legitimate for comparing

154

generalized situations at different periods of life but it gives no information on development because it does not study this. How different kinds of person change as they grow is not the same as how persons in general change, and only the study of history, which is development, can elucidate the former.

Beyond this, however, the study of history may be necessary for the inference of causal behaviour, for the person's present behaviour may be intelligible only if one knows how it developed from his past. If this is so, then causal laws are in a sense developmental laws and the study of causal behaviour and the study of development for its own sake are the same. Causal analysis depends on asking specific comparative questions, in the first place about the person's phenomenal or effective present. But this is not exactly delimited. It may go back only a few weeks or it may go back to the beginning of the present phase of the person's life (if that is more remote). In any case, it can be delimited only as a section of a continuous causal sequence. The decision to study only a short section of this sequence may be made on practical grounds, but on theoretical grounds it is arbitrary. Lewin's vague distinction [38, Ch. 5] between systematic and historical causes must be tested by reference to experience, and it may be noted that in another text his emphasis on the psychological field at the time as the cause of behaviour is qualified [39, p. 306] by the observation that long periods may have to be studied to determine the 'direction and velocity of behaviour'. However that may be, it is clear that the length of time one should study can only be determined by reference to experience. In order to understand a person's behaviour now, it may be necessary to take account of where he thinks he is going. Most psychologists, at all events, would accept the person's perception of and planning for his expected future as relevant to this kind of analysis. In the same way, it may be necessary to take account of where he came from, at the next move back, or the next, and so on. The possibility can be written off only if the laws of development are so firmly established that one can rely on similarities and differences in the present situation without further explanation. It follows from the argument of Chapters 6 and 7 that present similarities can only be similarities on a ground of ultimate difference where persons have different histories, as to some extent they must have. The question is whether ultimate differences are such that they can be ignored in the practical analysis of the present situation.

That this is unlikely may be demonstrated by the analysis of a case. There are two workmen, of the same age, engaged in the same trade, employed by the same firm and in closely similar economic circumstances. They have closely similar habits in their home behaviour, in social activities and leisure pursuits, and the same general outlook on society. Both intend to stay with their present employers as long as they can because they like their workmates and foreman as well as their work, although they are not very keen on the bosses and want higher pay. The prognosis for these two men is the same, that both will stay where they are, barring accidents; and their place in a general analysis of the behaviour of industrial workers is the same.

But their work history is different. One has had two jobs, including his present job, in fifteen years after finishing his apprenticeship and the other has had nine jobs in the same time, two (including his present job) of three years each and the other seven of an average length of fifteen months. The latter left his first eight jobs soon after he had quarrelled violently with the foreman, going of his own choice when he was not sacked. The occasions of his quarrels do not sound serious enough to warrant the energy he says he put into them. However, this is one possibility, that he was simply unlucky with his employers and that any man in his position would have got into a fight in the same way. If this is so, the difference between the histories of the two men is accidental and irrelevant to their similarity in the present. But the other possibility is that the rolling stone had a marked difference in the style of his job relations, a difference that would depend on his earliest social learning. This possibility is tested by exploring the upbringing of the two men, as they perceive it (independent evidence, let alone contemporary records, are of course unlikely). It is then found that one of them got on ordinarily well with his family while the other's relations with his father are best described as guerrilla war, conducted by him with some success from the age of 8 to 14, when his father died. One can then say that the one is normal and the other, the rolling stone, is an anti-paternalistic schizoid.

This may explain the past, but it leaves the present situation open. The one thing which is certain about this is that the two men are not in the same situation, but there are several possibilities for the rolling stone as compared with the settled worker. He may actually see his present situation differently, so that he may be expected to blow up and leave his job sooner or later. If he sees his situation in the same way (as far as the interview record goes) this may be because he finds it, at the moment, unalarming although he has not learnt how to manage his irrational anxiety. But then he does not see the situation in the same way. Seeing it in the light of his past experience, he sees it as a situation which is safe at last, though not altogether to be trusted; and he would probably see it in much the same way if his past experience had been due solely to bad luck in finding jobs where he was not well treated. The settled worker, of course, sees the situation in the light of his experience as just another good job, or a better, more convenient, more pleasant job. Or again, the rolling stone may see his present job as secure because he has learnt that he need not fight back at the slightest sign of hostility on the part of his foreman. The settled worker sees the same job as secure because the foreman is all right: which again is not the same situation.

One might be able to decide among these possibilities by investigating the workers' hypothetical actions. Asking them what they would do if they were transferred to another or to a somewhat inferior job, or if they were offered promotion, or asking them to state the qualities of a good job or a good boss, might elucidate their differences in perception of the present situation. So might questions about their expected future, if the job situation itself is likely to change. But, whether or not these methods were sufficient to define the difference in perception, there must be a difference (that is, one of several possible differences) because each worker sees his present situation in the light of his past experience.

If differences of detail (in attitudes to various aspects of the work situation, of other activities and so on) are finally detected, it could certainly be said that their cause is in the present situation. It is the person's perception of the whole situation (in the light of his past experience) which causes his differential perception of details. But this means only that the details are connected and coherent and can be summed up under a general condition: it does not mean that history can be written off either in the investigation or in the explanation of the present situation.

In the case taken, which is a fairly ordinary industrial case, it is not at all likely that the present situation of the two men could be adequately investigated without reference to their history. As first stated, the case may seem unreal, for no interviewer would be likely to find such close similarity between two men over a wide range of overt behaviour (including opinions, attitudes and intentions) unless they really were similar. That may be, though it is not unlikely that the first indication of a difference would be, as suggested, in job history, which the personnel officer relies on as a prognostic guide. But even if there are marked differences in perception of the present situation, these still have to be interpreted. A diagnostic test might show that one man is normal and the other schizoid, but that is not enough. No diagnostic test will show that a man is an anti-paternalistic schizoid who is specially liable to get into a fight with his boss for insufficient reason. Diagnostic tests may explain, but they can hardly predict, a historical style as specific as that. The interpretation may then be referred to the persons' recent history, when it is found that their records in their present employment differ significantly; or finally it may be referred to their general work history. This, and nothing less than this, would be sufficient for the investigation of the present situation. One could then say that the differences found are due to an apparently continuing difference in style between the two persons; or that they are the reflection in the present situation of similar styles that have been differently learnt; and so on. Exploration of the differences in present or past styles must of course be referred further back in history, as incorporated in the laws of development.

It is unfortunate that these laws are not sufficiently established to give an answer even to the particular question proposed about the two workmen. It is clear that the person's earliest social learning is relatively inaccessible to later modifying influences, so that quasi-infantile gratifications, narcissistic fantasies, excessive object attachment and so on may be expected in general to limit the range of adaptive adult behaviour. The successive definition of the person's behaviour has been discussed in general in Chapter 6, but just how it works in particular is little understood. This question can only be answered by the study of development; that is, of actual history. As already noted, cross-sectional studies are no substitute for this because they omit the connectedness of behaviour and so simply are not historical. History as the person now sees it, which Chein [11] calls the 'present past', must be accepted as a substitute and it may be possible to make some allowance for repression, distortion and condensation. Perceived history, as reported in the interview, may be backed up by critical hypothetical questions, by the indirect exploration of sub-intentional behaviour and perhaps by the enactment of critical situations; so that the methods of groups 4, 5 and perhaps 3 may support those of group 2. If this is done, it may be possible to determine the relation of actual to perceived history by systematic comparative studies of perceived histories only.

The other possibility is that the relation can be determined only by the direct comparison of perceived history with actual contemporary records. If this is so, the psychologist is for this purpose obliged to study a process on the same scale as his own life; he is thrown back on to real and continued acquaintance as a method of enquiry. This would be an irremoveable limitation of psychology as a set of methods of condensed acquaintance and would make the elucidation of the laws of development a lengthy task. The different possibilities here, however, do not affect the practical conclusion that a psychological enquiry into real life behaviour of any kind must in any case include an enquiry into perceived history if it is to end with a thorough causal analysis. Whether the laws of development are established by either kind of comparative study or whether they are in their present rather speculative form (depending on insufficient comparative study), they must be referred to, if only implicitly, not only to explain perceptions in the present situation but also to decide which perceptions are similar (in the light of similar experience) and which are different.

THE INVESTIGATION OF THE EXCEPTIONAL

Psychological enquiry, then, is obliged to go beyond present behaviour and to consider the duration of behaviour. In the same way, it may be necessary to go beyond common behaviour and to include within the scope of enquiry both behaviour which is not recurrent in the person's life and behaviour which is not found in a general class of persons. History already includes the former, for it is the history of events and not of phases or habits only. The latter would be included by a study of the singular or exceptional event, habit or person and would therefore be related to the study of history in so far as persons tend to singularity in their whole lives rather than in isolated actions or habits.

It may be as well to be clear that what is proposed is not really unknown to psychology. The singularity of the person, at least in degree, is accepted as an obvious empirical fact that needs no argument. In the most abstract analysis of behaviour, it is accepted that persons differ in their test scores, so that no two persons may have an identical set of scores if a large battery of tests is used, and no two summed scores may be exactly the same if regression weights are used. Or sets of scores may all be different, but some totals identical or of the same practical effect (all pass or fail). Again, the same total score may be derived from different collections of right answers, and the same pattern of right answers may be chosen by one person who works with a pen and another who uses a pencil. It is assumed that such differences are irrelevant because they are below the level of generalization that concerns psychology. Doubtless this is so, but it can hardly be assumed that all singularities are of this low order. The assumption would come oddly from a body of graduate professional workers who are as markedly singular in their ideas as is any other body of the same intellectual eminence. At all events, it is possible that the unimportance of singularity depends largely on the use of methods of enquiry that pass by the singular. Common experience suggests that functional equivalence, and therefore replaceability, are not altogether obvious even with relatively simple functions, such as doing unskilled factory work.

The functional equivalence of persons in more specialized jobs is far from obvious and in close personal relations it is hardly imaginable. This is another way of putting the point that persons tend to singularity in their whole lives rather than in the fragments that psychology often studies.

Whether or not there are, as common experience suggests there are, singularities of an order that is relevant to a general psychology, can be seen by considering what kinds of exceptional occurrence might be studied. Four cases are distinguished.

(a) *The single event.* There are many things that, in a sense, happen to everyone or that everyone does once only or rarely. The person's first job, his marriage, settling into a home and the birth of his children are events in this class. So are unemployment, bereavement and illness, and other common misfortunes. What matters about these best and worst things in the person's life is that they are likely to be critical events or turning points in his development, crises which radically change his perception and orientation. This possibility is perhaps more obvious with those events that begin a phase of life, but applies also to the others. In the study of real behaviour psychology has been largely concerned with the smooth level of recurrent behaviour in settled life phases, and has paid little attention to changes from phase to phase, let alone to other critical events. What needs doing here is to enlarge the study of the person's history so as to concentrate it on critical events and especially on critical changes as much as on habitual behaviour. Until this is done, the basis of the general laws of development must remain uncertain.

(b) *Behaviour under exceptional stress.* The effect of continuingly severe conditions of life on behaviour has been studied quite extensively, both where the stress is in the person's present conditions and where it is internal, due to earlier stress situations. The point here, therefore, is not so much to enlarge the scope of the enquiry as to change its balance. It appears, for example, that the most general reaction to severe deprivation is some kind of regression. Thus Sherif [61, Ch. 16] notes regressive behaviour in the inmates of concentration camps; Tinbergen [68, p. 208], writing of hunger from the zoologist's point of view, concludes that reason is: 'relatively weak when it is up against really powerful instinctive motivation'; and various writers have described how the unemployed family shrinks in on itself and tries to cut itself off from the world. But, however general these reactions are, they are not universal. There are records enough of persons who have risen to the occasion and maintained their integrity under conditions of severe physical deprivation or psychological isolation or both. On the first two points mentioned, Nansen's contemporary record [49] of concentration camp life has plenty of examples of exceptional, as well as of regressive, behaviour, besides being itself a striking example of the former. On the effects of unemployment, Bakke [3] and the Pilgrim Trust report [55] both note exceptional cases of adaptation as well as the general reaction. But it is the general case which has been studied, sometimes in considerable detail, and the exception, if it is noticed at all, is written off as a deviant.

A parallel with a difference of emphasis is found in the study of the endogenous stresses of psychoneurosis and psychosis. A great deal of attention has been given to studying and describing how the case goes from bad to worse in the natural course of events. The possibility that the patient himself may achieve a stable and even a socially well-adapted state by striving with his difficulties over years of tormented effort, until he finds a workable style, is noticed but hardly seriously considered. But this is how many persons handle their lesser difficulties, and some patients do the same. From the psychiatrist's practical point of view, the majority are deviants and may be fairly neglected, if not entirely ignored. As in the case of external stress, the effect is that the evidence is only partially studied. The question of the relevance of the exceptional case to a systematic psychology is prejudged by the decision that it is irrelevant: only particular study of the exceptional case in relation to the general can determine this question.

(c) *The singular style.* That there are persons whose behaviour is markedly 'deviant' in many areas of real life does not need demonstration. Allport refers to these persons [1, pp. 302, 303] as having individual traits that are hardly found in the general population. One could go a little further and say that there are persons whose patterns of traits or habits, or whose whole style, has no close analogue in the general population. These persons are usually disregarded in psychological enquiry.

(d) *The singular response.* This is the most limited case, as it includes only uncommon fragments in the behaviour of persons who are for the most part not uncommon. Some responses to projective tests, for example, would be classed here. Responses even to words, as discussed in Chapters 9 and 10, may be classifiable only if one includes a category of *different* individual responses (e.g. 'Book—to read at leisure, or study, to write is much better'); and the scoring of original responses in Rorschach records is well known. Equally individual behaviour may be found in real life, for example in leisure activities, as with the factory process worker whose hobby is hawking and falconry or the fireman whose spare time job is inventing complicated and mostly unworkable gadgets. Such behaviour is usually suppressed in a general analysis.

It is not suggested, of course, that any of the kinds of behaviour described must be strictly singular, except in the limiting and trivial sense that all general behaviour is singular. However, they are uncommon and they are, on the whole, disregarded by psychology because they are uncommon. The suggestion is that they should be studied as thoroughly as common behaviour is, because they are uncommon. The relation of uncommon behaviour to psychological law need not be discussed here, nor need it be asserted that such behaviour must be relevant to the analysis of particular cases. It is an important possibility, however, that particular enquiries would be assisted by taking the fact of 'deviant' cases and trying to find out why they are deviant; that is, by making a comparative analysis of kinds of common behaviour, not only among themselves, but together with uncommon behaviour. The possibility would depend on the case. It may be supposed that general but not recurrent behaviour (the single event, which is uncommon only in time) would be the most relevant, but behaviour under exceptional stress and the study of the singular style (which may well be related in some cases) might well be as relevant. The singular response is likely to be the least relevant because it is a fragment, but it should be as relevant as any other fragment.

A comparative analysis thus extended would at the least be able to explore the workable limits and social functions of both 'deviation' and conformity. It might also elucidate some particular problems, such as Sherif's puzzle [61, p. 453], of 'the unique individuality' of the creative artist and similar puzzles about other social nonconformists. Of course it would require a considerable extension of the evidence. It would be necessary to extend the enquiry into behaviour in real situations, to include situations which do not recur and which are exceptional in their nature; and to extend also to include persons of marked individuality. How far these extensions could be made simply by interviewing, backed up by the appropriate indirect methods, may be doubted. However, there would be no objection to including the autobiography (which seems to have been used only by Murray [48] in recent years) as a suitable indirect method, and this could perhaps be extended by the elaboration of special projective tests of a semi-biographical type.

In sharp contrast to the general neglect of exceptional behaviour is the attention paid to it in the one case where it is not likely to matter, in the use of abstract particulate tests. It is usual to consider the reliability of these tests as an important element in their results, and this means particularly, if not only, the reliability of performance of the persons who did them. The test situation is so handled that the person or group of persons are all set to undertake a task that they understand in principle and at which they are prepared to do their best. The question is then raised whether the person did understand the task and do his best, and especially whether there were marked differences between persons in these respects. From one point of view, it is a purely hypothetical question. The only exact definition of reliable performance is a performance such that the persons would repeat it exactly if they did the test again under identical conditions. This is not an operational definition, because they cannot do the test again under identical conditions; they cannot do it again for the first time. In consequence, the various conventional measures of reliability are inferential. The test correlates highly with itself, repeated, with a parallel version, within itself, and so on; whence it is reasonably inferred that the persons were all playing the game and nobody was playing his own individual game. The same inference can be drawn, of course, from a sufficiently high correlation between the test and anything else at all. It is possible that the rather low validity of the earlier cognitive tests (that is, their low correlations with each other, and with examination criteria and the like) was the point of departure for the separate consideration of reliability; for the hypothesis that the persons tested did not play the game may have seemed likelier than the hypothesis that the tests were unsuitable in nature in specifiable respects.

However that may be, the estimations of validity and reliability are now firmly established as branches of the higher statistics and great importance is attached to slight differences between the two figures and between the figures for different tests. This approach unfortunately obscures the only point that matters; that reliable and valid performances are not properties of the test but particular historical facts. The certificate of good character and the certificate of proficiency both show what the test has done under particular conditions, not what it will do under any conditions. The conditions for validity require systematic study and, strictly considered, those for reliability do also. The most rigorous procedure would be to estimate reliability after each use of the test and report that it was (not is) satisfactory. It might be sufficient to rely on inference from previous known conditions of testing to new testing situations; but, in practice, not even this is necessary. The conditions under which performance is unreliable are known to every experienced tester and are simple and obvious. The test may be too hard, however it is introduced, so that the persons tested are almost non-starters and flounder at random after the first few items. The detailed instructions about the task may be insufficient, so that some persons do the wrong thing. If the test is well chosen and introduced, there may still be some persons of little intellectual sophistication who are scared of it and who are therefore non-starters, or who adopt an inefficient style of work in a strange situation and bolt through to the end of the test regardless of the quality of their performance. Lastly, it does happen that the persons tested simply do not want to do their best; for example, the rifleman does not want to be re-trained as an anti-tank gunner and sees to it that his scores disqualify him. All of these difficulties except perhaps the last can be surmounted by a good tester, if only by the desperate measure of using a conversational individual test (Binet or Bellevue) instead of a group test. All, equally, should be obvious to any but the most incompetent tester when they have occurred in a testing session. For practical purposes, the possibility that the persons tested were out of step with each other or with the tester or both can be disregarded. As a general problem it may well be worth investigating, but the matter to investigate would be under what conditions of work, with what tests, do different kinds of persons accept the idea of doing their best, understand what they have to do and set about it as efficiently as they can. In such an investigation of common and not singular behaviour reliability coefficients would play only an accessory part.

THE EXPERIMENTER'S INTERVENTION

If the individuality of the persons investigated by the psychologist may need special consideration, it might none the less be expected that his individuality does not. The experimenter has the same basic training as other experimenters and similar experience; he works together with others and discusses procedures and results with them. Everything is done to ensure that experimenters, as such, are interchangeable. However, it can hardly be assumed that they are completely so. How far they may be expected to be will depend not only on their community of personality, training and experience but also on the stage of the enquiry, from framing hypotheses through to formulating conclusions. It is hardly possible to consider all these stages, but the intermediate stages of gathering and handling data merit attention.

In their administration, methods of enquiry range from the fool-proof routine of the abstract test to the individual relation of the open interview. There is hardly any room for variation in the actual enquiry or in the recording of results with the abstract methods or with the indirect methods, except perhaps those of group 3. With the interview and perhaps with the staged situation more variation is possible. It may or may not make a difference to what the person says that he expected to be interviewed by the professor and was interviewed by a mere research assistant, or by a man instead of a nice girl, as he expected. Whether or not it does will depend partly, at least, on the interviewer's perception of the situation and ability to handle it. Beyond this kind of difference, which may be irreducible, there may also be personal differences among experimenters, who may be specially good at interviewing young workers or children or adults generally or maladjusted persons, and not so good at interviewing the other kinds of person they necessarily encounter in the course of the enquiry. Recording reported or observed behaviour is probably open to little variation provided that a uniform procedure is adopted. The best procedure is probably to record as much as possible as it happens or is spoken, for this is less open to hurried on the spot interpretation than are procedures that openly depend on interpretation, such as rating schemes and pre-coded survey variables.

Individual variations in the handling of data are probably more to be expected. There can be none, except plain mistakes, in the stencil scoring of abstract tests. Some may occur with tests that are scored by example; that is, in the use of a content analysis. A simple case is the vocabulary items of the Binet test; a more complex one the scoring of a Rorschach record. Most variation is probably found in the use of those methods (chiefly the interview) with which the experimenter must make his own content analysis in all cases. The same would apply, of course, to the first content analysis of a set of projective test records. Even with interview material, however, it seems likely that variations would be much less if the content analysis is made after the interviews (categorical abstraction alone) than if it is made during the interview on a pre-arranged rating or coding scheme. This may be expected even if the scheme (which is an example of instrumental definition) is derived from a thorough empirical content analysis of other interviews, which is not a usual procedure.

It may be concluded that reducible differences between experimenters, or differences other than those imported by the persons' reacting differently to different experimenters, may be found both in the recording and in the handling of data. The former kind of unreliability, however, is easily reduced by adequate recording methods and the latter, whether or not it can be reduced, does not appear to be very serious. There remains the possibility of reducible differences due to the experimenters' different handling of the situation. These, as noted above, would matter only with the interview, but how much they would matter, and under what conditions, are

M   165

open questions. Some findings that bear on these and other questions may be briefly mentioned.

In the course of an industrial enquiry, a hundred workers in a factory were interviewed. The interview was open, with a fairly complex check list and usually took an hour or more. For various reasons, it was necessary to do the work quickly, so that thirteen interviewers took part in it. They had much the same background of training and all had some experience, but there were marked differences in the closeness with which they were able to work with the person who had prepared the check list and who directed the interviewing. On the basis of these differences, the interviewers divide into three groups: the supervisor alone, who conducted a quarter of the interviews, then seven persons who did an average of eight interviews each, then five who did an average of three each. Analysis of the records shows a three per cent loss of information in the records of the second group as compared with those of the supervisor and an eleven per cent loss in the records of the third group. These losses derive from reducible differences between interviewers (for irreducible differences would distort but not omit information), and include differences in both handling and recording the interview. The larger is not a serious loss and it occurred under conditions of work that would be acceptable only for special reasons. It may be concluded that under orderly conditions of work (adequate training, full briefing, ample time for discussing progress and full recording), the unreliability of interviews is not a serious consideration.

Variations in making or using the content analysis of a projective test do not seem considerable either. The validities of the six projective test items discussed in Chapters 9 and 10 are relevant evidence. They show that the analyser must have been consistent throughout his work, so that this could presumably be repeated by other experimenters working under the same conditions. Agreement between scorers of Rorschach records (cf. Cronbach [15, p. 437]) shows that variations in the use of a content analysis made by one person are inconsiderable. These findings, of course, relate to empirical content analyses: it is not to be expected that they would hold where categorical abstraction is applied.

It is worth noting, however, that uniformity in the handling of data seems to depend more on orderly conditions of work than on the experimenter's making a full and explicit content analysis. The marking of school examinations, for example, could be regarded as a reduced content analysis, made at a high speed with the aid of some categorical abstraction. It is often supposed that this is an unreliable procedure but some of the evidence which is usually quoted to show this shows, on the contrary, that the procedure is reliable under specifiable orderly conditions. It would be out of place to enlarge on this point, which has been sufficiently discussed elsewhere [52, pp. 149–153]. Its relevance is that, with regard to the long standing and vexed questions of the reliability of school examiners as well as with regard to the consistency of any other assessors of psychological data, what needs investigating is not merely the statistical estimate of their performance but under what conditions they are or are not consistent. The simplest answer to the problem of the personal factor in psychological enquiry is to include differences between experimenters as part of the data to be analysed in all cases. Where the data have been gathered or handled or both by more than one person, the persons concerned are a logical part of the investigation. They may indeed be the main point of the investigation, which can as well be directed to study how judgements are made, and under what conditions they are sound, as to studying the content of these judgements.

This is a point of some importance, because of the wide use of synthetic judgements in psychology. It is implied in the general account given of methods of enquiry that any summary findings about persons or groups of persons will be derived step by step by a rigorous analysis of the data. This is a reasonable prescription for general enquiries conducted by trained persons under no pressure of time. In other circumstances it is not reasonable. In applied psychology, for example, the clinical diagnosis, the interview appraisal of suitability for employment or the assessment of suitability for promotion from observation of a role-playing series, must proceed directly to a single practical judgement which classifies the person. This may be called a synthetic judgement because it synthesises all the evidence by one swift process which the judge may be unable to analyse, let alone communicate to others. Much the same kind of judgement is made by non-psychologists who are asked to act as raters or assessors generally in psychological enquiries.

It seems to be generally thought that synthetic judgements are both disreputable and unreliable because the judge cannot say how he makes them. The evidence hardly supports this idea. Eysenck's analyses [20, 21] of check list diagnostic items and of the test performances of persons diagnosed as neurotic or psychotic, show that the psychiatrists who made the initial diagnoses on which his experiments depended were reasonably consistent in their work both between each other and from time to time; for, if they had not been, there would have been only specific factors (or unreliability) to extract from the analysis. In the case quoted from Cronbach [15, p. 397] which is mentioned in the discussion of the methods of group 7, in Chapter 9, it is likely that a synthetic judgement instead

167

of a fragmented one would have been quite reliable. MacIver observes [41, Ch. 5] that defining marital maladjustment as that quality which causes a close friend to rate a couple as maladjusted is meaningless unless one knows the basis of his rating. His objection is met in part by the fact that scales for measuring marital maladjustment (and many other such operationally defined phenomena) have sufficient internal consistency for it to be inferred that they are measuring something coherent. Showing that the close friend was not merely guessing does not, of course, show just how, and on what grounds, he made his judgements, and this applies to the other two cases quoted. It is hardly possible to infer the composition of a synthetic judgement from statistically related items as abstract as scores on psychophysical tests. However, the inference is easy in principle, as it depends only on the analysis of the material used in the judgement or of information from direct or indirect methods which can reasonably be transferred to the judging situation. McClelland [40, pp. 99, 100] reports a case of the former kind, in which the inference could have been made. The analysis of Thematic Apperception and word-association test items discussed in relation to the methods of group 5 in Chapters 9 and 10 shows the possibilities of both cases. If a complete analysis showed sufficiently close relations between scaled responses and the synthetic judgements of members of the selection board (as it probably would), it should be possible to infer, both how the projective tests were used in making some judgements and, by analogical transfer, how the other judgements were made from other material.

These cases, of course, are only indications for full investigations, but they are sufficient to show that there is something well worth investigating. Synthetic judgements need not be abandoned because they have been shown to be unreliable. Naturally, the wider the range of investigation the better. Examinations and fully developed methods of enquiry should both be included, and an enquiry into the internal economy of psychoanalysis (which could be done quite easily by a content analysis of records) would probably be useful. All of these investigations would have the two aspects mentioned above. As investigations of what is recorded, categorized, interpreted or judged they would be general enquiries relevant to the elaboration of psychological laws of general behaviour. As investigations of the processes of recording, judging and so on they would be instrumental enquiries, from which special laws of behaviour might be derived. The results would certainly suffice to dispose of the silly controversy about intuitive and scientific judgements by demonstrating the nature of the trained guessing which bridges the gap between these two supposed extremes. The results should also be sufficient to simplify the practical procedures of the various fields of applied psychology and perhaps to simplify the methods of general enquiry.

At all events, the limits of variation due to the experimenter's intervention would then be known. Meantime, one can only rely on the indications that these variations are slight in the worst case. It may be expected that they would be greatest with the most complex and least communicable methods of enquiry, such as psychoanalysis and the ordinary open interview (as well as some merely inefficient methods, such as trait rating and graphology, the complexity of which is due to instrumental definition or categorical abstraction). Personal variations in indirect methods of enquiry are probably less and in abstract methods are hardly possible. Of course, even if these suggestions must be relied on for practical purposes, it is still important to take particular notice of variation between experimenters in any actual enquiry where this can be studied separately. In principle, this is yet another addition, though a very slight one, to the mass of evidence necessary in psychological enquiry.

A general conclusion about the three extensions of the evidence that have been discussed is simply stated. The point of all three is that psychological enquiry is obliged to go beyond the simple scheme of generalizable behaviour or quasi-universals studied by a detached and impartial observer, to include the study of the person's concrete historical individuality by another individual. The historical and individual (which are ultimately one) must be taken into account and neither dismissed as trivial nor shunned as unmanageable (because of 'unreliability') in a scientific investigation. The three extensions suggested are of course of unequal importance. The inclusion of history is much the most important, and perhaps not very much open to doubt on the ground of reliability. The inclusion of the exceptional (so far as it does not come in with history) is important and little, if at all, open to doubt. The inclusion of variations between experimenters is the least important, but should be made because variations certainly occur. All three kinds of evidence, then, should be taken into account; and this means that they should be both incorporated in or allowed for in the findings of the investigation and taken into the formulation of psychological laws.

THE NATURE OF LAW IN
PSYCHOLOGY

THE argument has now traversed a wide area, in successive stages of definition. The field of psychological enquiry is defined by the inclusion within it of all empirical and communicable propositions about the behaviour of persons, and not of certain classes only of supposedly privileged propositions. The matter to be investigated is described by reference to the person's concrete historical engagement in his world, and the methods of investigation are compared in detail, in relation to the scope and nature of the evidence required. The obvious next step is to consider what happens after the investigation, in the formulation of psychological laws.

This means returning to the conclusions about hypotheses in psychology and considering the distinctions between general and component hypotheses, on the one hand, and between real and abstract hypotheses, on the other, in the light of the discussion of how to get what kind of evidence, for what purposes. Hypotheses can now be considered as laws, for the two are continuous with each other in any science. Stevens [66, p. 27] says: 'Science, as we find it, is a set of empirical propositions agreed upon by members of society.' If this statement is meant to define the status of scientific knowledge, it is doubtful; and it would be entertaining to pursue the implications of the last six words in the statement. However, as a historical proposition it is perfectly sound. In the history of science there is an orderly progress from the wild speculation to the sober hypothesis, the established law and perhaps finally the discard of superseded theories. Dobereiner's law of triads never got beyond the first stage, while Mendeleyev's classification of the chemical elements has long been in the third and the phlogiston theory is safe in the discard. From the historical point of view, then, a law is merely a hypothesis that has become respectable by being admitted to good society. Law and hypothesis in psychology are of the same kind or kinds and the discussion of either stands for that of the other. The discussion is undertaken after the detailed analysis of methods of investigation because this is its place in the logical sequence. The psychologist speculates or proposes a hypothesis, decides his general methods for testing it and the range of behaviour to which they are to be applied, gets his data, analyses them, draws conclusions and formulates either a law or another hypothesis. The final product, of course, is the beginning of the next sequence and it is immaterial what it is called so long as it is discussed in its place, as the final product of a sequence. It is proposed, then, to state a hypothesis (or speculation, if the lesser dignity seems more fitting) about the nature of law in psychology, in the same way as Chapter 9 states a hypothesis about methods of enquiry and the whole book states a hypothesis about psychology.

THE GENERAL CHARACTERISTICS OF LAW

In any field of knowledge, not only in the natural sciences, a law classifies phenomena in some kind of ordered series from which deductions can be made. The law is an inductive generalization of any kind from observed phenomena and it is assumed that the classification the law sets out would hold for identical phenomena that have not been observed. This assumption may not be logically justifiable. Wisdom [72] argues that it is not, but concludes [72, Ch. 24] that making the leap in the dark is perhaps likelier to be right than not making it. Collingwood [14, pp. 254, 255] more robustly asserts that, while there is no logical compulsion to make inductive generalizations there is a conventional virtual compulsion, the legitimacy of which is guaranteed by theology. At all events, there is a practical compulsion to generalize, as there is to assume the necessary connections of causality, in order to undertake an intelligent ordering of life; and this may be taken as sufficient ground for the generalizations of psychology.

The phenomena classified may be things as they are seen or events or processes that are not directly heard or seen. The psychological law, of course, classifies together abstracted processes that are thought to have important general properties in common. That these processes are apprehended little, if at all, by the use of external physical instruments gives the law no special status, for the generalization and naming on which it depends are formally equivalent to those which produce the abstractions of scientific laws (e.g. heat, energy, ionization, nervous impulse). The ordered series of the law

171

may be any kind of series in which the relations of the members can be unambiguously stated: quasi-physical series and series of other mathematical types are admissible but can claim no special status.

The most important characteristic of a law is that deductions can be made from it. This means predictions, in a carefully limited sense, so that prediction is the same as explanation. Marx [44, Ch. 1] distinguishes the two in stating that explanation and not prediction is the business of science. The confusion here is probably because psychology aims to explain behaviour generally (like a science) while applied psychology may be called upon to predict what an individual will do in specified circumstances (like a technology). As long as the circumstances are carefully defined, however, there is no incompatibility, for explanation is prediction in hypothetical and general circumstances. The circumstances specified in a psychological law are hypothetical as they are applied in deduction for, strictly, the exact circumstances in which the initial observations were made can never repeat, as the person in history is singular. It must be allowed, of course, that this limitation may not affect deduction if the singularity of the person is at a trivial level of behaviour with which deduction is not concerned. However, the circumstances and behaviour specified in the law would usually be so generalized and abstracted from actual singular cases that they may be expected not to repeat exactly for any single case or even for any general group of cases. Thus exact prediction in any actual case, particular or general, may be impossible but this does not detract from the law's exactness in hypothetical prediction. Further, the relations specified in the law may be approximate only even in the hypothetical case; and deduction is then probable (within specifiable limits) but not certain even in hypothetical circumstances. This too does not affect the standing of the law.

It may be likely that the practical prediction which is required in applied psychology, even as this tends towards being the art of understanding the singular, can depend to a reasonable extent on general laws, in so far as hypothetical circumstances are approximately reproduced in the particular case. But it is not necessary that this should be so for a law to be accepted as sound. A law is a summary of experience, not a prophecy. It is accepted as a sound summary if it meets the minimal requirements outlined: that it is based on observed phenomena, the relations among which are exactly described in a general form which can be applied to hypothetical identical cases.

In approaching the discussion of the characteristics of laws that go beyond the minimal requirements, it may be as well to note that these do not include brevity and simplicity, which are to be regarded as convenient incidental features of a law that has them rather than as necessary or even desirable features in any sense. A law of any complexity is, in principle, as capable of satisfying the minimal requirements as is a simple one. Hypothetical prediction, or the precise deduction of consequences in identical cases, requires that the law is unambiguously stated, so that identical cases are clearly defined. For this purpose, a psychological law may require several books to state rather than a few lines; but so long as the statement is unambiguous, it has exactly the same standing as the elegantly simple mathematical law. One must allow, indeed, that a psychological law is likely to require a long and complex statement. Besides clear definition in the statement of the law, precise deduction requires that the law should be applicable over the whole range of phenomena from which it was inferred (not beyond this range: extrapolation, as it is called with physical laws, is another question). This requirement can be met only inferentially, for no law is tested over the whole of a continuous range. However, with physical laws the difficulty is not serious, for it is a little unlikely that a law of this kind would apply to the tested parts of the range but not to intermediate parts: e.g. that Boyle's law would hold for ten observed pressures from 0·1 to 57 atmospheres, but not for pressures between those observed. In psychology, however, one is more likely to be concerned with discontinuous series of qualitative classes, such as personality traits, occupational groups, diagnostic classes and so on. Interpolation in a series of this kind is hardly to be attempted, so that the law must depend on the making of some observations in all classes. It follows that a law of any generality is likely to require a long and complex statement.

However, a psychological law can be of very little generality. The minimal requirements, in fact, would be met perfectly by a very restricted component law that was so specialized that it could hardly be transferred by analogy to any similar case and so localized that it could be expected not to hold for any length of time. An example is the finding that bearded vegetarians prefer the works of Bernard Shaw to those of Aristophanes. This specimen of nonsense is entitled to rank as a law. Taking the three observed cases of persons with the characteristics stated, it generalizes from them the phenomenon of literary preference in a series of two exactly defined-classes: and the consequence can be deduced that the odds on the preference of the next bearded vegetarian one meets are such and such. The law is unfortunately limited in that it states nothing of general relevance anyway, nothing that could be expected to apply to beardless carnivores, and nothing that could be expected to hold beyond the duration of the fashions for beards, cabbages and Shaw. None the less

173

it is a perfectly sound law. The minimal requirements of soundness are of no relevance to the usefulness of the law, so that the three main conditions of the latter must be considered separately.

CRITERIA OF USEFULNESS

A useful law is firstly one which is *broadly applicable* in hypothetical circumstances, and not applicable only in narrowly specialized areas of behaviour. This recalls the distinction between component and general hypotheses, a distinction in a continuous range. However necessary it may be to start with laws at the limited end of the range, usefulness obviously increases as these laws are summed through the range. Secondly, therefore, a law which is *broadly applicable by analogical transfer* is more useful than one which is not. A law, like a hypothesis, states what persons do what kinds of thing under what circumstances. It may be expected to be approximately applicable to slightly different persons, behaviour and circumstances if it is not too narrowly specialized. This application may be necessary because it is all that can be done in areas which have not been investigated, and the investigation of such areas is itself facilitated by the analogical transfer of laws for other areas, which enables the easy formulation of hypotheses and the development of component into general laws. Lastly, a useful law is one that *may be expected to hold for a fairly long period of time*. This may seem a difficult condition, for psychological laws are necessarily historical. They state, not what has been observed in a universe which does not change in historical time and what may therefore be expected to hold through history, but what has been observed in history and may be expected not to hold as soon as society has changed appreciably. Nobody would expect that the same laws about job expectations, the perception of social classes, marriage and the family or neuroses, for example, would be equally valid for the Byzantine Empire, medieval France and seventeenth-century Scotland. But there may be changes that are within the scope of psychology. The laws of psychoanalysis, for example, were derived largely from a period in which and a locality where sexual and excretory behaviour were regarded as particularly shameful. They were always of doubtful applicability to primitive societies of the same period, and it seems likely that their validity elsewhere has already been reduced by changes in modes of bringing up children. Psychology cannot, of course, get ahead of history by prophesying social change and a law which, in the extreme case, referred to hypothetical circumstances that were no longer found would be perfectly valid. It would be more useful if it made some provision against possible or probable change, as it could do by enlarging its scope. In the case suggested, the laws of psychoanalysis were derived largely from the study of the patriarchal family, which seems to be much less common now than it was fifty years ago. These laws would have been less open to attenuation by change (if this has indeed happened to them) if they had derived from the equally systematic study of other kinds of family; and this could have been done quite easily as other kinds were found, not only in primitive societies, but also as exceptional (and therefore neglected) cases in European society. Further, a law's probable life may be affected by the kind, as well as the range, of the data from which it derives. Some verbal cognitive tests and personality questionnaires include items that date fairly quickly because they refer to narrowly localized events or verbal customs or social habits, whereas the data of direct and indirect methods of enquiry are less open to this kind of ageing.

It may be concluded that a law is likely to be durable if it has a wide scope and depends on unspecialized data, so that broad applicability in time depends on the generality of the law as much as does broad applicability in range, whether directly or by transfer. Thus valid laws, which all satisfy the minimal requirements, may differ widely in their usefulness or economy, and it is these differences that must be discussed in relation to the main types of law. The types may be classified by reference to distinctions in the three main features of psychological laws.

1. The kind of behaviour which the law summarizes. This may be *ordinary* behaviour in real life situations of all areas, including self-directed behaviour and including sub-intentional and intellectual behaviour in real life. Or it may be *abstract* behaviour, in constructed situations for which there is no analogue in real life. This distinction corresponds to that between the direct and indirect methods of enquiry on the one hand (so far as the results of the latter can be transferred to real life situations), and the abstract methods on the other hand.

2. The kind of series which the law states. This may be *causal*, in the historical or systematic sense, in which case comparative differences in intentional perception are traced back to sufficient differences at the beginning of the sequence. Or it may be *classificatory*, describing concomitant events and variations without referring to intentional perceptions. This distinction corresponds to that between the methods of group 2, with its accessories in groups 3 and 4, and the methods of the other groups. It also corresponds to the distinction between data

175

that have been as little abstracted as possible in analysis and data that have been put through the three processes of abstraction described in Chapter 10.

3. The form in which the law is stated. This may be *direct*, in plain language, with a limited use of special words and of statistical definitions. Or it may be *mathematical*, depending on the analogy with the physical dimensions and stated in the terms of parametric statistics. Or it may be *analogical*, stated in the terms of other mathematical analogies (such as topology) or of dramatic or biological analogies. The distinction between direct and mathematical forms also corresponds to that between unabstracted and abstracted data.

These distinctions, of course, are not sharp and absolute, but it will be convenient to treat them as if they were in the following discussion of the main types of law. It should be noted that the examples given in this discussion are meant only to be sufficient to demonstrate the features of the type, not to be finished statements of laws. In some cases they could not be finished statements anyway, for only an invented law (that is, a hypothesis or speculation) can be stated at the present. In any case, it has not been thought necessary to set the examples out in full, for some at least would have run to the length of a book if this had been done.

ORDINARY CAUSAL LAWS, DIRECT OR MATHEMATICAL

An example of laws of this type may be taken from abnormal psychology. Persons who habitually indulge in exuberant mendacity (described in full, together with other hysteric behaviour) see themselves as rejected by the persons they love (and so on, in detail), while in unconscious fantasy they re-enact certain (detailed) parental attachments, in consequence of the relations (described) of their infancy and childhood; whereas compulsives, schizophrenics and manic-depressives . . . (the sequence of overt behaviour, perception, sub-intentional behaviour and historical origins in learning is repeated in detail for each case). Another example may be taken from social psychology. Persons who are striving for advancement in their occupations see themselves as obliged to get ahead in the face of competition, in order to secure their self-esteem and in consequence of their identification with the systems of personal values taught them in school and urged upon them by their fathers; whereas persons who are not so striving do not see themselves as obliged to secure their self-esteem in this way, in consequence of their either having rejected their fathers' urgings or having not been subject to them.

These are examples of fairly general laws, which could easily be broken up into, or built up from, various components. Thus the first might be reduced to a comparison of hysterics with all other persons together, or to comparisons among hysterics, distinguished by sex, phase of life, occupation and so on. The second example could be reduced similarly to comparisons among occupational climbers distinguished] by class (employed, self-employed and so on). On the other hand, both laws could be made more general by extension to include observations made in other societies or, of course, by combination, in a form which compared manics who are striving for success with compulsives who are not, and so on. The following argument applies equally to the laws as stated and to the reduced or enlarged forms.

These laws are valid, as they satisfy the minimal requirements for this. That both are inductive generalizations (or summaries of observed events) is obvious. They arrange phenomena in a series in the sense that they order, by conceptual abstraction or generalization, certain kinds of recurrent behaviour which are classified according to their resemblances and differences in the whole sequence from past to present. How this is done depends on the question of what one means by recurrent behaviour, which, with a number of related questions, is much too large a question to discuss here even if it were within the scope of the argument. It may be taken that it can be done and, once it is done, the definition of the phenomena and of the ordered series in direct language (as far as this is possible) or in a mathematical form is equally valid.

In this respect the direct and mathematical forms of the ordinary causal law seem not to differ, at least in their unambiguity. The borders of events and classes of events are determined by the communicability among experimenters of their definitions. Statistical analysis (of data about real behaviour, of course) is doubtless necessary both to trace the relations between events and to clear the ground in the definition and serial ordering of events. But, following the argument of Chapter 10, this analysis should be empirically conservative rather than parametric; and it seems likely that the actual statement of the law need not go beyond a similar conservative use of statistics. The possibility, at all events, can be traced with reference to the undefined terms in the examples of law set out above. It is necessary, of course, that such terms as hysteric, striving, identification, rejection and so on, should be defined operationally, for unless they are defined in terms of the procedures used to isolate them they are not defined at all but are merely ambiguous. But there are many possibilities here. Hysteria, for example, might be defined by the single answer to one critical question, if a suitable indirect (group 4) question could be found. It might be defined as an exactly specified combination of real life behaviours, which themselves would be defined by the instruments used to investigate them. Or it could even be defined by a range of patterns (not sums) of projective test responses. All these definitions would be established by statistical analysis, perhaps including parametric methods, but the latter would not be included in the definitions. The case in which this was done (the mathematical law) would depend equally on real life behaviour investigated by any appropriate method, but analysed by scaling; that is, it would depend on data that had been confounded by addition in a case where this was psychologically unnecessary.

This does not affect the precision of the hypothetical mathematical law, which is as unambiguous as is the directly stated law. The latter may be somewhat easier to understand (communicate) as its statements about real behaviour are more direct; and, if this is so, it would also be easier to deduce consequences from the directly stated law. However, these differences are not considerable and there would be no other differences between the two kinds of law in the possibility of deducing consequences from them. They are equally likely to allow of occasional ambiguous cases, whether by overlapping classes or anomalous factor patterns; and equally likely to specify a degree of statistical approximation (e.g. the law holds for eighty-six per cent of the cases observed).

It may be concluded that an ordinary causal law which is stated as far as possible in direct language, with only the most conservative use of statistical definitions, is as likely to satisfy the minimal requirements of validity as is a law stated in the terms of parametric statistics. The conclusion is important, for if the mathematical statement, which is fashionable with other types of law, especially the abstract type, is to be introduced into laws of the ordinary type, it must be justified on other grounds. Economy of statement (a few equations instead of a lengthy description) is not a sufficient ground, for equations have to be interpreted by reference to a description of their content anyway. Greater usefulness, or breadth of application, would be a sufficient ground; but the more an ordinary law tends towards mathematical statement the less useful it is, in the sense defined above.

This is to be expected on general grounds, apart from the consideration of the usefulness of the ordinary law in particular respects. The mathematical form of statement requires the statistical abstraction of data about real life behaviour, and it has already been argued that this abstraction, together with the processes that precede it, is very likely to confound the natural order of the data to such an extent that both the inference of intentional perceptions and the transfer of findings to real situations are rendered difficult or impossible. If striving, self-esteem and identification with the father's values, for example, are reduced from summary descriptions depending on the person's connected report to correlations between job attitude, personal evaluation and paternal esteem scales derived by abstraction from the same material, both difficulties are likely. But then the mathematically stated law is not an ordinary causal law at all. Depending on how seriously the data are confounded, it becomes an ordinary or an abstract classificatory law; and both of these are much more limited in their general usefulness and applicability than is the ordinary causal law.

The conclusion that the mathematically stated ordinary causal law is inferior in principle, if indeed it can retain its status at all, is important because ordinary causal laws conservatively stated are more useful, in the sense defined at the beginning of the chapter, than are laws of any other type. They are obviously of broad application, as they refer directly to real behaviour and for the same reason they are capable of application by transfer to other situations. Knowing the nature and origin of occupational strivings among self-employed persons, for example, enables one both to make a fair guess at the differences to be expected among employed professional workers and to develop the exact investigation of these differences more readily. Such knowledge might even enable a fair guess in what is a contrasting rather than an analogous situation, that of the employed artisan or the unskilled worker. The same kind of transferability would hold for the first example given above; e.g. among schizophrenics of different ages, social classes or societies or, as a contrasting case, of different sex. Finally, the broad scope of the ordinary causal law and its derivation from connected real life behaviour makes it more durable than laws of other types.

The discussion of ordinary causal laws began with two examples of historical laws of overt behaviour in areas of real life. This is not the only kind of ordinary causal law and some other kinds need to be distinguished, as the conclusion that ordinary causal laws which are stated as directly as possible are the most useful applies to them also.

The ordinary causal law which is not historical may be considered first. This is a law which omits duration but retains intentional perception as cause. In its least form it may be a mere tautology. Thus it could be said that schizoids are sometimes openly aggressive and sometimes quietly dreamy because they want to be, or that persons who do or do not strive to advance in their occupations do or do not want

179

to advance. These statements include only the universal proposition that persons do things because they want to, which, as a universal proposition, is not open to comparative analysis. The statements are therefore not causal, although they are quite sound as classificatory or descriptive laws of little generality. However, this is the least case, and both statements are easily expanded into comparative analyses. The schizoid is openly aggressive where he sees a threat to his self-esteem and sits back dreaming that he is the universal emperor where he sees no threat. Some persons strive for advancement in order to secure their self-esteem, others in order to secure peace at home and others in order to secure an early retirement and go fishing. These simple and superficial statements are comparative analyses, of differences between occasions and persons respectively, and what they state is a sufficient immediate cause of these differences, a cause which is not given in the mere statement of the differences nor, indeed, in common experience. They break up a part of a non-causal classification into intelligible sub-classes which are distinguished by differences in intention; and of course they could be extended to do the same for the rest of the classification.

These statements are therefore causal laws, of the sort that Lewin [38, Ch. 5] calls systematic, as distinct from historical. This distinction is of minor importance, both because it is drawn within ordinary causal laws and because it is, on the whole, arbitrary. The systematic law certainly applies to only one phase of a sequence, but this is not timeless; for the habitual behaviour on which a law of any generality depends must be observed in the extended effective present. The connectedness of behaviour can be sectioned at any convenient point, and sectioning to include only the effective present may be convenient but has no other claim to preference among causal laws. The systematic law enlarges into a historical law by the simple addition of remoter sequences in order and becomes more and more general as it goes back. It may be regarded as the limiting case of the ordinary causal law in one direction, while the historical law which goes back to birth is the limiting case in the other. Continuity in the range does not depend on the curious idea that the past is effective in the present but simply on the repeating sequence from cause to effect, from effect as cause to the next effect and so on. Where in this range the line is to be drawn will depend on a compromise between the generality but tedious derivation of the historical law and the easy derivation but limited applicability of the systematic law. The latter is not only capable of enlargement, it positively invites it; the description, for example, of present differences in the intentional perceptions of persons who are striving for advancement is somewhat superficial unless these differences can be explained.

The ordinary causal law, then, is systematic instead of historical if it refers to events of short duration. Reference to behaviour which is generalized from all areas of real behaviour instead of being specified separately for each area may also produce a systematic law. The second law stated above refers to behaviour in the specific area of work, as well as inner personal behaviour. The first example does not distinguish between specific areas of real behaviour (e.g. home, work, social activities) as it is set out, though it probably would if it were set out in full. As set out, however, it is a historical law because it refers to kinds of generalized behaviour which are linked directly to causal situations. The case with generalized classifications of adjustive techniques (Cameron [7, Ch. 6]) or defence mechanisms (Fenichel [23, Ch. 9]) is different. These classify behaviour which is abstracted from, rather than which simply occurs in, all areas. Withdrawal and regression, as described by Cameron, for example, are general classes of behaviour as compared to the social specificity of striving for advancement or mendacity. Such general classes of behaviour cannot be directly linked with past causal situations, because each may have several different kinds of cause. Both withdrawal and regression are associated with various kinds of present behaviour (that is, are used by persons with different kinds of specific total maladjustment) and are derived from different kinds of early causal situations. Classifications of such behaviour therefore cannot be historical laws. In so far as they imply perceptions which are not obviously given in the situation (e.g. the person sees himself confronted with a task that cannot be done without lowering self-esteem and cannot be avoided, and therefore develops a severe headache), these classifications are ordinary casual laws of the systematic type. If there is no such implication, they are not causal laws at all but classificatory.

The last point to be noted about the ordinary causal law is that it need not refer to overt intentional behaviour. The first example given above includes, and the second implies, sub-intentional behaviour ranging from conscious wishes to unconscious fantasies. Such behaviour may be overt, at the extreme where it is coherent enough to be hardly distinguishable from formulated intentions, and can therefore be reported if the person is prepared to do that: or covert because the person is not prepared to report or, with unconscious fantasies, because he cannot. If sub-intentional behaviour in ordinary real life situations can reasonably be investigated or inferred, it can be the content of an ordinary causal law by itself. The law can be historical, stating that persons have such and such recurrent fantasies because of the way they perceive their present situation, in consequence of their upbringing. If the last term is omitted the law is of the systematic sub-variety, but if only the first is stated (a description of kinds of recurrent fantasy in real life situations) the law is not causal but classificatory. The case with intellectual behaviour in real life situations is not so clear. If it is sustained, it may be possible to detach it from the intentional behaviour which is supports. For example, the person's planning of a long continued project for advancing himself in his occupation might be taken by itself, though its separation from the execution of the project would be distinctly artificial. However, if it were so taken, the planning could presumably be analysed in detail so as to relate each elaboration to the person's perception of its function and its place in the whole scheme. For example, he decided not to use his acquaintance with his boss's daughter as an entry to his boss's social circle because that would involve him in more time than he could spare from certain other sub-projects. If such analyses were made extensively, it might be possible to incorporate them in an ordinary causal law of the systematic variety. Extension into a historical sequence is hardly conceivable and reduction to a classificatory law (including only what was done in the planning) is perhaps likely.

ORDINARY CLASSIFICATORY LAWS, DIRECT OR MATHEMATICAL

Laws in this class refer to behaviour in ordinary real life situations but not to the person's perception of these situations or to the origin of his perception, so that they are not causal. Examples have already been given in the discussion of the reduction of causal laws by the omission of perceptions; and further examples may be added. A description of the overt behaviour which is characteristic of the different kinds of neurosis is a classificatory law, for it specifies what goes with what and how patterns of related events are to be distinguished without stating the immediate causes of these patterns. A classification of types of family organization is a classificatory law if it depends only on who does what, and not on how the members of the family see their activities and relations. Lastly, a classification of types of job, depending on the activities of persons engaged in different jobs, is a classificatory law.

In principle, the classificatory law can always be enlarged into a causal law either by the direct inference of perceptions or by further investigation. The examples given would differ considerably in practice, however. Direct inference might be possible with family data (the unco-operative child is one who sees himself as rejected), but the classification of neuroses could be enlarged only by further investigation, as the relation between what the neurotic says he does and why he thinks he does it is often by no means given in what he does. Enlargement of a job classification is, of course, beyond the scope of psychology. The cause of the division between the doctor's and the dentist's professions may be an accumulation of intentions to specialize the treatment of patients, as the cause of the difference between the guillotine operator's job and all others may lie in someone's perception that this machine was needed and could be made; but these causes belong to sociological history, not to psychology.

However, whether or not the classificatory law of ordinary behaviour can be converted into a causal law of psychology, it is a perfectly valid law. It satisfies the minimal requirements for validity in the same way as the ordinary causal law does. On the other hand, it is less useful than the causal law even if it refers to the same areas of real behaviour. As it explains less of the behaviour in these areas, it is more likely to be only approximately applicable. A correct diagnosis of a patient (which is a deduction from the general laws of neurosis) is easier if one knows what neurotics do, in relation to the way they see their situation, than if one knows only the former. The person who copes with a job which is too big for him, but which he dare not leave, by confining himself to the meticulous execution of the trivial routine parts of the job may be a schizoid who has struck an uneasy compromise between trying to live an impossible fantasy and fleeing; but, if one knows only what he does in the job, he may appear to be a compulsive. It follows that the analogical transferability and the durability of the classificatory law are less than those of the causal law. The transfer of a classification of family organizations or of neurotic syndromes from one social class to another may involve misapplications due to class differences in superficial customs, in the division of work in the household, for example, or in the person's frequency of recourse to the family doctor. If the law includes a statement of why the housework is divided as it is, or why the doctor is or is not consulted on such and such occasions, misapplications in transfer are less likely. Durability is subject to the same reservation. Fashions in symptoms, for example, change quite quickly enough for classifications of syndromes without perceptions to require revision from time to time. An example is bad night vision, which was a very popular symptom in the early part of the last war and is now almost unknown.

The difference between the direct and mathematical statements of the classificatory law is much the same as it is for the causal law. A mathematical statement of an ordinary law, about behaviour in real life situations, can be made only by the confounding of the natural order of the data. It has already been argued that this process may be taken far enough, with causal data, for the causal law to be reduced to a classificatory one (if perceptions can no longer be inferred). If the process is taken to the limit, as in the statistical addition of naturally ordered elements of various jobs or of neurotic syndromes, what would have been an ordinary law, whether causal or classificatory, becomes an abstract classificatory law, as job scales or neurotic factors can no longer be referred to real situations. The limiting case in the other direction is that the mathematical statement of a classificatory law is taken only just to the point where reference to real behaviour can still be made. This hypothetical kind of law would be only a degree less useful than would a law stated in direct terms with the least possible use of quasi-physical measures and the two might, indeed, be hard to distinguish. The important point here, as with the causal law, is that the direct statement is more useful, however slightly in this case, and equally valid, and is therefore to be preferred.

In conclusion, the point may be repeated that the laws of subintentional and intellectual behaviour in real situations, as discussed above, are perhaps more likely to be classificatory than causal.

ABSTRACT CLASSIFICATORY LAWS

These are the ordinary classifications of empiricist psychology. Neuroses and psychoses are classified by scores on abstract diagnostic tests, jobs by psychographs, job aspirations and job satisfaction by inventory scores, family organizations by adjustment scales and so on. Such classification of behaviour which is mostly referred to the present (it cannot be called present behaviour in the ordinary sense because it is behaviour in the test situation only) can be extended to include reference to past behaviour. One example will suffice: the correlations between children's scores on home adjustment scales and their scores as adults ten years later on job and marital adequacy scales are such and such.

These laws are abstract in that they refer to behaviour which occurs only in the test situation. The examples given would derive, wholly or largely, from the abstract methods of group 7, which include items that do refer directly to behaviour in real life situations. But all these references are fragmentary and they are unconnected even with each other, so that even if they are references to specific real behaviour (which is not often the case), they do not refer to that behaviour as it actually occurs. Laws derived from the methods of groups 8 and 9 (of which examples are not given) are even more obviously abstract, as much or all of the behaviour they refer to (e.g. analysis of diagrams or number series or mechanical puzzles) does not occur in real life in any form at all.

It follows that these laws must be mathematically stated. Addition is the only possible process for summarizing the results on which they depend, and a statement in direct language could only expand into words the mathematical formulas which state the summarized results (norms, correlations and so on). These formulas, of course, must be backed up by a direct statement of their derivation, but this merely describes their terms (e.g. z in the equation is the total score on such and such a scale). With these laws the mathematical statement is appropriate, then, simply because it is the intended summary of the whole investigation.

Laws of this sort are necessarily not causal, as MacIver [41, Ch. 3] observes, because they cannot include intentional perceptions. Of course, it can be said that persons score on a personality inventory or on an aptitude test because they perceive the task, to varying extents, in the way the experimenter intended them to, but this is a mere tautology. The inference of comparative differences in perception between tests can be made in the same way but must be equally a mere tautology unless the difference is pursued, by inference backed up by introspection, into performances on single items. Even if this were tried, it is doubtful that the inference could be made and an analysis of this kind never would be done (except in order to derive a law of method, as described below) because the whole point of using abstract methods of enquiry is to infer laws of real behaviour. If an abstract law is transferred, by analogy, to ordinary behaviour, intentional perceptions can be inferred just so far as the transfer is reasonable. Thus it could be said that scores on an introversion scale depend on how far the person perceives himself as brilliant but unpopular (and so on through the whole range of scoring responses) in real life. However, this is really a tautology also, because it merely states that real life perceptions are directly reflected in the test performance, and does not connect these perceptions with behaviour which is derived from them but not closely similar. In any case, that direct reflection can be assumed is very doubtful, as will be argued in the discussion of the usefulness of abstract laws.

A specious substitute for causal inference is the statement of a statistical relation in abstract laws that refer either to related tests or to the relation between a test and some classification of ordinary behaviour. Many statistical relations, or correlations, are of a low order, so that one can only infer from them that the correlated variables have something in common but not very much. If the correlation is high (as it is between fairly similar abstract tests, and only in this case) it is certainly easier to describe what it is that the variables have in common. Even with perfect correlation, however, as Césari [10, pp. 203–220] argues, causation has to be inferred on other grounds. The inference is doubtless easier but in this case as in others the possibilities that A caused B, that B caused A and that C caused both are not discriminated by the mere fact of correlation. Thus far the argument is on common ground. The point is easily missed, however, that it is irrelevant because it refers to physical and not intentional causation. A score on a family adjustment scale does not cause a score on a job adequacy scale, whether these are contemporary or separated by ten years. Neither does family adjustment, transferred to real life but abstractly defined, cause job adequacy similarly treated. What causes a person to be adequate in the performance of his job is his perception of the requirements of the job as relevant to his personal goals (an ordinary causal law of the systematic variety), where his present personal goals originate in his perception of his family's values as relevant to his earlier purposes (a historical law). Now the intentional perceptions stated could, of course, be identified as the elements A and B, or A, B and C and so on, in the causal analysis suggested above. But they cannot be identified with any credibility from abstract measures. It is not the failure of the correlation to discriminate possibilities that prevents causal analysis, it is the abstraction of the data and therefore of the law, to which process the correlation is merely incidental.

It must be observed, too, that there is no short cut to causal analysis through the intervening variable, as described by Marx, Spence and Tolman [44, 64 and 69 respectively]. Given that family adjustment and job adequacy are highly correlated as test scores or, by inference, in reality, one can explain the correlation by saying that family adjustment causes job adequacy through identification of the boss with the father, or that both are caused by a general trait of social conformity. These new variables could certainly be operationally defined and their relations tested, so that the original abstract law might be enlarged by the investigation of further hypotheses. If this were done, it would still be an abstract classificatory law, for the inference of intentional behaviour in ordinary situations is as likely to be made more difficult as it is to be facilitated by the accumulation of abstract measures. If the intervening or supervening variables were taken as explanatory and not further investigated (which is a common procedure), the only addition to the original abstract law would be an elegant labelling of the experimenter's ignorance.

The abstract classificatory law, then, is incapable of conversion into a causal law, not because it is classificatory (the ordinary classificatory law can usually be made causal) nor primarily because it must be mathematically stated, but simply because it is abstract.

This is naturally even more marked for the law as applied by analogy to ordinary behaviour. However, this in no way invalidates it as a law. It is an inductive inference depending on phenomena in a serial order, both of which are strictly operationally defined. In these respects it is no worse (and no better) than any other kind of law. Deductions can be made from it and in the simplest case these are precise. One can say exactly (with specified sampling errors, that is) that x per cent of an identical population tested with scale A will exceed a score of twenty, and so on. Where the law specifies a relation (the correlation between A and B, for example), one can again say exactly that x per cent of an identical population tested with both scales will exceed a score of twenty on A and seventeen on B. However, these exact deductions are trivial. The deduction which is usually required is that of B from A, and this is likely to be more approximate than are such deductions with laws of other kinds.

This point leads directly on to the consideration of the usefulness, or applicability, of the abstract law. It has no direct application at all. There is no question of its applying to any area of real behaviour directly and its direct application as an abstract law, as in the trivial cases outlined above, is of no use whatever. Except perhaps in the underworld of applied psychology, nobody wants to know how a person stands in relation to other persons on some abstract measure just for the sake of knowing that. The information is meaningless. Equally, nobody wants to deduce a person's score on one test from his score on another test and go no further, for the deduced score by itself is again meaningless as well as markedly approximate.

The only possible use of the abstract law is in analogical transfer to behaviour in ordinary real life situations; the use for which substantially abstracted measures are constructed (as the easiest means of condensed acquaintance) and abstract laws derived from them. It hardly needs to be repeated that abstract laws which include abstract measures and ordinary classifications of real life behaviour (e.g. discrimination between occupational groups or psychiatric diagnostic classes by test or inventory scores, correlations between tests and examinations) are known to be of a generally rather low order of precision. Where the analogical transfer depends on an unknown relation it is likely to be even less precise, especially where the transfer is made directly to real life behaviour. For example, a neurotic inventory discriminates significantly but not much more than that between persons rated as normal and those rated as neurotic, whence it is inferred that the inventory scores are useful indicators of persons' competence in conducting their daily affairs. Or it is inferred from the correlation of 0·65 between an intelligence test and some school examinations that the test is a useful indicator of socially effective intelligence or real intellectual behaviour. These inferences from abstract to real would be doubtful in any case and the approximate relations on which they may be based do not so much support as throw more doubt upon them.

It may be concluded that abstract classificatory laws are much less useful than ordinary classificatory laws and still less useful than ordinary causal laws. This is a conclusion of the first importance, because abstract laws are almost established as the typical laws of psychology as a science. Whatever the reasons for this may be, their known and repeatedly demonstrated weaknesses are sufficient to annul their claim to a special status even though laws of other types are comparatively very little developed. The abstract law depends for its usefulness (not for its validity in the limited sense) on a transfer by analogies so remote that one could reasonably place the onus of proof that the transfer can be made on those who wish to make it. In a good many years of work, no proof has been produced but many poorly approximate transfers have been reported. It seems reasonable to assume now that the addition axiom on which abstraction depends is false. If one begins work with a heap of broken bits of masonry, timber, piping and tiles, one can certainly arrive at a tidy set of sorted heaps by systematic work; but this set is no more a building than is the original heap. Whatever uses the abstract law may have, it cannot substitute for ordinary laws any more than can its disreputable cousin the magazine quiz (on Are you a real person? etc.), the disreputability of which derives much more from its abstract nature than from its mere lack of statistical sophistication.

LAWS OF METHOD

The chief weakness of the abstract law, that it cannot be referred to behaviour outside the test situation, may be turned to account if it is referred deliberately to comparative differences of behaviour in test situations, when it becomes a law of method. Chapter 9 is an example of an elaborate hypothesis that might reduce to a law of this type, or break up into a number of such laws. A simpler example may be taken from projective testing (the methods of group 5). Projective tests range considerably in their definition of the response, from story completion tests in which the end is almost defined by the text given, through stories about pictures, sentence completion, word association and the Rorschach test, to a hypothetical extreme in which the person is observed while aimlessly doodling. The behaviour they elicit may be referred to the person's ordinary conscious or unconscious behaviour and may be articulate or fragmentary. The hypothesis is that the behaviour elicited follows the range in definition, from brief, conscious and articulate but stereotyped behaviour with the most defined, to extended and fragmentary behaviour derived from the person's unconscious fantasies with the least defined; so that articulate behaviour derived from unconscious fantasies may be elicited, if at all, as a sort of compromise in the middle of the range of tests.

Similar hypotheses, or potential laws, could be proposed for differences between methods in groups 7, 8 and 9: e.g. differences in performance between several neurotic inventories or several tests of mechanical aptitude. All these, if they were established as laws, would be abstract laws because they would refer only to behaviour in the test situations, compared with each other. Not all, however, would otherwise resemble the abstract classificatory laws which are referred by transfer to ordinary behaviour. It should be possible to infer differences in intentional perception of the method of enquiry, over the whole range of methods from direct to abstract; that is, differences in the way the person sees his purposes as related to the experimenter's, through the medium of the method of enquiry used. If such differences can be inferred, or established by particular enquiry, the law of method is an *abstract causal law*, of the systematic variety. This might still be possible with the hypothetical law of projective tests, but would be doubtful with laws of method confined to abstract methods, for with these sharply defined tasks it would be hard to establish any differences in perception beyond those that were obvious in the test material. It might be expected, then, that a limited abstract classificatory law would remain classificatory if it were turned into a law of method.

It would be quite appropriate to state laws of method as directly as possible. Projective tests, for example, can be ordered by inspection of their results, if not of the tests themselves, with regard to their definition of the response expected; and this ordering would be sufficiently defined by a list of tests, without the use of an elaborate statistical measure of definition.

Laws of method obviously satisfy the minimal requirements of validity and indeed, if they refer to abstract methods, are more likely to do so than are abstract laws referred to ordinary behaviour. The latter reference is analogical and approximate, while the abstract law of abstract methods is directly applicable and may be highly exact. The range of applicability of laws of methods is, of course, narrow; but they have important uses in principle both in guiding the selection of methods of enquiry and in the elaboration of new methods. A new projective test, for example, could be interpolated in the

189

existing range if the law of this range were established; or a new projective interviewing technique could be developed if a law including both direct and indirect methods were established. The durability of laws of method may be open to doubt; but it could be said, on the whole, that the use of the abstract law, which is irrelevant to real behaviour, lies here in the summary handling of methods of enquiry.

THE LIMITS OF LAW IN
PSYCHOLOGY

THE discussion of law in psychology has been directed so far chiefly to the distinction between ordinary causal laws and abstract laws; and the conclusion is that the former are appropriate for ordinary behaviour and the latter are acceptable as laws of method. This suggests limits to the kinds of law that are possible in psychology, and certain other limiting features remain to be discussed. Before this is done, however, it may be as well to observe that the major distinction made in Chapter 12, sharpened as it is for the purpose of exposition, obviously depends on what one means by ordinary behaviour.

In Chapter 8, and thence through the next three chapters, ordinary behaviour is rather taken to mean recurrent behaviour in long connected sequences, especially behaviour with persons. This is not meant to imply, of course, that there is no other ordinary behaviour or none of importance, either to the person himself or to the psychological observer. In particular, the person's engagement with things, as studied in work on visual perception in various modes, hearing, attention, fatigue and so on, has been little noticed. For the person, this is obviously a very important set of engagements, and its importance is duly reflected in the attention given to it in psychology, from the earliest days of experimental work up to the latest developments in 'human engineering'. That it has been adequately attended to in psychology is the reason for its omission from the preceding account (apart from a few references in Chapter 9); but it would be misleading to leave it at that. This is the field in which scientifically designed experiments and the use of physical measures are appropriate. In this field there is no question of the transfer by analogy of abstract laws to ordinary situations; for, with this special kind of sub-intentional behaviour, the experimental situation can obviously stand for the ordinary situation. As the objections to abstraction in other fields depend on the illegitimacy of arguing from one situation to another quite unlike it, they do not hold in this field, in which abstract laws are quite legitimate.

The distinction between ordinary causal laws and abstract laws stands for all fields of intentional behaviour, and may now be generalized somewhat by considering the question of how the law is stated. The distinction between direct and mathematical statements of laws is incidental to the distinction between ordinary causal laws and abstract laws; for the latter depends on the content of the investigation, and therefore the law, while the former distinction depends only on the kind of language used. Now mathematics is a special language, highly developed, complicated and abstracted, which contains only logical propositions; that is, highly elaborate definitions which have no necessary application to any events at all. Any application of mathematical language to things or processes or classes of events is to some extent an application by analogy or metaphor. In its classical phase, mathematics includes propositions about number or quantity, abstractly conceived, and this language may be fairly directly applicable to events in some fields. It has been suggested that the analogy, or metaphor, of quantity is not obviously relevant, or is probably irrelevant, to many fields of human behaviour. What remains to be considered is other possible analogies.

ANALOGICAL LAWS

It may be said at once that the statement of a psychological law in plain ordinary language is likely to be the clearest and most precise form of statement, provided that all the terms are defined (as far as may be necessary, statistically). As Allport [1, p. 340] suggests, it may be much easier to use common words than to invent new ones; and, as Collingwood suggests [12, pp. 205, 206] for a similar purpose, it may actually be an advantage to use common words provided that their changed significance is clear from the context, as well as from particular definitions. At all events, this seems a likelier method of exact communication between experimenters than is the invention of new words (cf. Cattell [9, Ch. 21]), for the meaning of the law which refers to something already known, only known more clearly, is better conveyed by words which are already known. This is not to say that the occasional use of metaphors is undesirable. Any metaphor which the experimenter finds useful in clarifying or in communicating his ideas is quite legitimate, so long as it is clear that it is used only as an illustrative metaphor. Here again, however, the esoteric metaphor, like Eysenck's [21, Ch. 8] breaking stresses of metals, is less likely to be useful than the long-established range of poetic and dramatic metaphors, which may be equally far-fetched but are much better known.

The sustained use of metaphors, however, has no obvious advantages. Lewin [38] finds that spaces, regions, barriers, vectors and valences are useful concepts, so that one must allow that he found they aided his thinking. Their relevance as general aids to exposition is not obvious. Lewin's examples are no more than elaborate restatements of quite simple facts in a special language supported by complicated abstract diagrams. It seems, indeed, that the elementary topology which he uses amounts only to a few classical syllogisms about inclusion and exclusion, that could be stated more simply in their usual form in texts on logic than they are in the topological form. This special mathematical language does not appear to be any more useful than is the conventional statistical language of quantity. It is quite possible, of course, that some variety of the special language of mathematics may be found to offer a unique exactness in the formulation of psychological laws. However, this is an empirical or historical question. If a particular condensed and symbolic language would be advantageous, the likely way of determining this is to develop the shorthand of psychology in its own right on the basis of formulations in plain language. At all events, this would be a likelier procedure than the borrowing of someone else's shorthand, whether that of the biologists or physicists or that of the more recent pure mathematicians.

Meantime, it can hardly be accepted that the relatively abstract metaphorical shorthand of topology has any advantages. That some of the facts reported by Lewin are important experimental findings merely increases the irrelevance of the mode of statement, because this has to be translated back into plain language anyway and the translation is the harder where the content is to some extent new. The same kind of objection applies to the consistent use of dramatic and sometimes biological metaphors by the psychoanalysts. This is a somewhat esoteric metaphorical shorthand, although it is not symbolic. One might argue whether the analysts' persistent use of this language, which seems to have been invented on the basis of the jargon of the medical schools of central Europe in the eighteen-nineties, has done more to facilitate the general acceptance of analytic theories by persons who mistakenly think they understand them than it has done in preventing the integration of analytic theories with psychology at large. However that may be, it is at least likely that some of the difficulties of analytic theory, and especially of the relations between theory and particular findings, would be capable of attention, if they were not explained, by the translation of their heavily metaphorical statement into plain language.

The popularity of metaphors in psychology is probably due to, or interdependent with, the tendency to look for laws of processes and not of persons. To say that the person is an intersection of forces, for example, opens the way immediately for the description of these forces while the person is forgotten. However, this metaphor, which is the one on which abstract laws using parametric statistics rely, is as legitimate as any other provided it is useful, in the sense described at the beginning of Chapter 12; and its accessory uses in defining terms have already been discussed.

A special case of the analogical statement of a psychological law is the application to human behaviour of the laws of animal behaviour. In themselves, these laws are perfectly valid, as ordinary or abstract laws (derived from observations in the species' natural environment or in the laboratory) of animal behaviour; and they might be further distinguished as causal or classificatory, depending on one's view of intentional perception in animals. However, these niceties can be left to the zoologists. As was argued in Chapter 3, the importance of this case is in the loose tendency to write of laws (of learning, neurosis and others) which have been established solely for certain animal species as if they applied, without further consideration, to persons. It is precisely because this is only a loose tendency, which is not uncommon in the more elementary psychology texts, that the point is important. Obviously there is no objection to the formulation of a law which has been found by investigation to hold both for animals and for persons. But the transfer of findings established on animals only is the likelier to be accepted for its being made only implicitly; and it is no more than an irrelevant analogy.

In this analogy, it is stated, in effect, that the person is a rat, dog, ape, protozoon and so on, who behaves according to the laws established for the animal species. But this is as much an analogical statement, depending on a zoological metaphor, as in the statement that the person is a mass of steel, intersection of forces, stage of a farcical tragedy and so on through the various metaphors. The basis of evidence, of course, is very different in the two cases. It is observed that persons behave in such and such a way, and the metaphor is brought into the statement of the law in order to clarify it, without any explicit or at all events any detailed reference to the observed behaviour of the metaphorical object. In the zoological metaphor, the detailed observations are of the animal and the person's behaviour is related, if at all explicitly, only on the basis of common experience. But this merely makes the metaphor more doubtful. The person is not to be regarded as a rat because it has been established that he behaves like one; he is to be regarded as a rat regardless of the evidence (if any), and therefore it will be asserted that he behaves like one.

THE LIMITS OF LAW

The discussion of types of law in psychology is, in effect, simply a discussion of different but equally possible psychologies. Laws of ordinary behaviour may be either causal or classificatory (the latter enlarging into the former, in principle), and require conservatively direct statement. Abstract laws are necessarily classificatory and are appropriately stated in a mathematical form. They are fully as valid as ordinary laws but, except for abstract laws of method (which may be causal), there is no relation between the two kinds. Abstract laws have no considerable application to ordinary behaviour and the mathematical (abstracted) form of the ordinary law would therefore be merely an uneconomical hybrid.

But this means only that the end of the enquiry depends on its beginning. The kind of law derived at the end depends on whether or not the data were abstracted in analysis, before that on whether direct, indirect or abstract methods of enquiry were used and before that on whether ordinary (real) or abstract hypotheses were proposed; and the whole enquiry depends in turn on whether or not the person's concrete historical engagement with his world is kept in view, which again depends on the initial wide or narrow view taken of the limits of the empirical proposition in psychology. It might be too extreme to say that there is an irreconcilable difference between a psychology of abstract laws and one of ordinary laws, but decades of work on the abstract have shown very little transferability to ordinary behaviour. The two can certainly not be regarded as interchangeable and the limitation of abstract psychology to the field of abstract behaviour is not only a present fact (as Marx [44, Ch. 1] notes), it is probably a permanent fact.

The boundary of the science of psychology, then, can be drawn so as to include abstract behaviour only or so as to include this (for what it is worth) together with ordinary behaviour. The latter case, however, presents a difficulty of another kind. If it is possible to establish ordinary laws that are for general purposes sufficient for the science of psychology, they will not necessarily be sufficient in the sense of inclusive. It may not be possible to explain all kinds of behaviour or, more particularly, the behaviour of all persons in hypothetical circumstances by means of general laws. Approximation in the application of a law depends simply on the lack of similarity between the behaviour it summarizes or the persons it refers to and the behaviour or persons (not circumstances: these are allowed to be hypothetical) to which it is applied. Deriving exact laws for all kinds of behaviour is therefore only a matter of time, until all kinds have been studied. But deriving exact laws for all persons may not be only a matter of studying them all, if that were possible. Lewin's view [38, Ch. 2] of the lawfulness of the individual case implies the simpler view, which McClelland [40, pp. 89–94] states, that a general law can always be applied to the individual case if this is studied closely enough.

However, it does not follow that it can be applied exactly and without residue. It is a fact within every practising psychologist's experience that some persons fit much worse than others into various general laws and Sherif's puzzle [61, Ch. 17] about certain striking 'deviants' may mean no more than this, that there are persons to whom general laws do apply only approximately, however carefully the case is analysed. Following the argument of Chapter 11, -this would not be a surprising finding. The extensions suggested there, in the deliberate study of 'deviants' as contrasting cases, as well as for their own sake, could easily be taken into the scheme of ordinary laws in some ways. If particular extensions or modifications of general laws are sufficient to accommodate the deviant cases, there is no problem. If these processes are not sufficient, it might still be possible to propose general laws of the variety, degree and effectiveness of exceptional behaviour or the exceptional person.

At this point the boundary of a psychology of ordinary behaviour may be reached, for the explanation of deviant cases may require individual laws, one for each person. It is true that this would be a quite logical extension. A psychology of ordinary behaviour would include laws of all behaviour, and laws applying to some kinds of behaviour in some societies, localities or groups of persons. The extension would therefore be only to state the individual law, in terms of the person's own history, which explained whatever of his behaviour in hypothetical circumstances could not be explained by more general laws. This kind of law, as Stephenson [65] has shown, can be as conventionally statistical as may be required, though presumably, as an ordinary causal law, it would be better stated in direct language. In any case, and whether the behaviour it explained was a small residue or was the greater part of the person's life, it would be only a step removed from the least general laws of ordinary behaviour.

The alternative is to exclude the law of the single case from psychology as a science. There is no objection to drawing the boundary here, as long as it is not implied that what lies beyond the boundary is not knowledge (because it is not science) and therefore must be ignorance. The boundary would be drawn, not between knowledge and ignorance, but between general (or conceptual or essential) knowledge and particular (or concrete) knowledge of being. As Gilson [26, p. 286] observes, the latter is prior:

'L'erreur fondamentale des métaphysiques de l'essence est de prendre la partie pour le tout et de spéculer sur l'essence comme si elle était l'être. Les essences ne devraient jamais être conçues comme les objets ultimes de la connaissànce intellectuelle, parce que leur nature même les engage dans l'être réel concret.'[1]

As psychology is obliged to consider, not only the single person under actual conditions (which is beyond the scope of science anyway), but the deviant case as much as the typical, it can do so quite simply by accepting the possibility of understanding the deviant as fully and as truly as it understands the typical. This means only that psychology is the art of studying being (the singular existent) as well as the science of the universal (or abstract essential). In so far as psychology follows life, it must be both. The science of psychology can be defined so as to include both or so as to exclude the art. Which is done is immaterial even to the applied psychologist who must practise both for, if the line is drawn on paper, he can ignore it in practice. With regard to this limit, the choice is not between this or that kind of psychology, it is merely between different limits of psychology as a science.

The question of formal delimitation, then, may be unimportant; but the evident fact that some persons fit poorly into the general laws of psychology may be of importance. Collingwood [14, pp. 148–150 and 177, 178] argues that historical causes are unique conjunctions of events and strongly objects to the formulation of general historical laws which depend on superficial and inadequate analogies between events. MacIver [41, p. 377, and generally] also rather suggests that the causal conjunction of large-scale events is unique. For events on a sufficiently large scale, such as the rise of the European nations, the assertion of uniqueness is likely enough; for, within the brief scope of history, there hardly could be anything more than a forced parallel. However, Collingwood may exaggerate, in practically suggesting that general analogical laws of history are impossible; and the question for events of any scale is ultimately empirical. The uniqueness of the person may be found to be a trivial residue or it may be found to be important. The point is that it

---

[1] 'The fundamental mistake of essentialist metaphysics is to take the part for the whole and to speculate about essence as if it were being. Essences should never be thought of as the final objects of intellectual knowledge, because their very nature engages them in real concrete being.'

cannot be assumed to be trivial, or to be merely an effect of the present insufficiency of psychological laws. Wherever the limit of psychology as a science is drawn, psychology as an applied art must allow for the possibility, if not the probability, that what lies beyond the scope of general laws may be important.

In other respects, the limits of psychological law hardly need special consideration. Differences between experimenters might have the consequence that the exactness of application of some laws was reduced by the difficulty of communicating them exactly, but this is hardly a notable point as it is evident that the study of persons is somewhat more complicated than the study of things. Finally, it is equally evident that the ultimate kinds of behaviour are beyond the scope of psychological laws, which can summarize comparative differences but not universals. That all persons strive for specified different things, and why their strivings differ, could both be taken into laws. But that they strive is simply a primary given fact; it could be explained only if it could be contrasted with the behaviour of persons who never strive for anything at all.

CONCLUSIONS

It is, indeed, possible that the ignoring of the singular existent is the origin of the confusion in psychology about the nature of law and, underlying this, the confusion about methods, hypotheses and basic presuppositions. The first necessary step in psychology is to compare persons by abstracting from their singularity, and this may lead to an unnecessary and rash second step in which the persons are dropped and abstract essences (such as ideology, aspirations, dominance, leadership, intelligence, ego, id) are compared without reference to persons. Psychology has then done the same as an established science, which studies abstract processes, and may then take the third and equally unnecessary step of setting up quasi-physical measures. It is not suggested, of course, that psychology has actually pursued the glittering promise of being a science like physics. But psychology is properly called a science in the sense in which any systematic body of knowledge is a science, and it is worth noting that this does not mean at all the same sense as with the natural sciences. Indeed, there is no reason why it should unless one holds that one type of law can include all natural phenomena, a view which, as Césari [10] argues, is demonstrably false.

No scientific laws are causal in the same sense as are psychological laws, for they are at least hypothetically independent of the person even as an observer. It might be said that Avogadro was the cause

198

of Avogadro's hypothesis, but he can hardly be identified as the cause of the phenomena stated in his hypothesis. The laws of the natural sciences are either simple discontinuous classifications or mathematical laws of process which, in effect, state infinitesimally continuous classifications. Thus in physics there is the table of specific gravities or Boyle's law; in chemistry, the periodic classification or the law of mass action; in physiology, the description of the three types of mammalian muscle fibre or the statistical laws of the relation of the respiratory quotient to the composition of food eaten, or of the heart's speed and stroke volume to its temperature; and in zoology, the general classification of animals or various physiological statistical laws.

The simple classifications of the natural sciences are not closely analogous to those of psychology. Classifying simple visible existents by easily defined features or easily measured processes, as in the taxonomy of zoology, gives results that are not entirely unambiguous, as Césari [10, pp. 135–142] shows. Presumably this is because animals are not easy to classify. It is then the less likely that the classifications of psychology, which include much more complex processes, for the most part apprehended by analogical self-reference and not directly perceived, could be either simple or entirely unambiguous. A likelier analogy is with philosophy, the classes of which, according to Collingwood [12, Ch. 3], may overlap because they include events (concepts) which are not simply one-dimensional and cannot be made so. Much the most reasonable analogy, of course, is with common experience. Collingwood elsewhere [13, p. 7] observes that psychology can only state (one must add, more clearly) what everyone knows, so that its depending on common experience for its classifications would be not so much a use of analogy as a simple return to its source. However, there is probably little attraction for psychology in the simple classificatory laws of the natural sciences.

This is not so true of the laws of mathematical process of the natural sciences, which might be thought to be causal laws of an exactness beyond the dreams of psychology, in that they specify concomitant variations which can be reproduced even under actual conditions with great precision. That is so: but they are not causal laws at all in the psychological sense. Psychology has no use for physical cause and effect laws of concomitant variation, not only because of the difficulties of deciding which caused which, but also because no uniform relation can be asserted which is independent of perception. The law is simply not a causal law until, as MacIver [41, Ch. 14] argues, it can refer by imaginative reconstruction to the person's dynamic assessment of the situation. Whatever it may be in nature, in psychology cause is intentional perception, so that the correct analogy for psychology is not with the natural sciences at all but with history. It was the lawful and traceable convergence of many intentional perceptions that led, for example, to the fall of Rome and of Byzantium. Neither was overthrown by an earthquake, any more than the person who falls into despair is merely pushed over by an external force.

The analogies on which psychology properly relies are not drawn from the natural sciences, then, but are found within its own field. The analogy of the person with himself at other times may be the closest, as it underlies the study of his recurrent behaviour, or, if extended, it may be outside the field of psychology as a science, when it is applied to the singular person. Psychology can then rely on the analogies between persons, which is its proper study and beyond which it need not go. The analogy of the person with an animal, an object with physical dimensions or a mathematical abstraction is remote enough to be of doubtful use even as an illustration and is quite irrelevant in the laws of psychology. Ryle [58, pp. 319–327] may be correct in holding that psychology is merely a fortuitous collection of enquiries. At all events, it is distinguished from psychology as everyone knows it by the specialization of its outlook and hence of its methods of enquiry and its laws. But the way to develop it into a science is not at all to assimilate it to the more obviously and quite differently specialized natural sciences, but to secure its special extensions of common experience firmly to their origin in common experience.

It may be noted, in conclusion, that the prospects of development in this sense rather depend on the school of psychology. The work of the social psychologists could be developed, where it is already inclined to phenomenal analysis and has a fairly wide cover of areas of behaviour as well as tight operational definitions, until it takes its natural place simply as psychology, instead of a special branch of it. Those parts of social psychology which depend rather on the abstract analysis of factors in social behaviour are no more open to development than are other empiricist enquiries, though all these, of course, can be elaborated indefinitely in detail by the construction of further and further abstract situations. The development of psychoanalysis in new fields is already proceeding, but would probably be faster and more communicable if its archaic language were abandoned and some attempts at operational definition (perhaps even backed up by the analysis of records) were made. The development of animal and physiological psychology are both open possibilities though, of course, on their own level only; neither, after however long a development, can ever relate directly to common experience.

THE SOCIAL INVOLVEMENT OF
PSYCHOLOGY

THE consideration of possible developments in the main schools or trends of psychology leads naturally to the consideration of the place psychology has made for itself in the world of knowledge. It is not necessary to consider the normative implications or social applications of psychology, and it would be beyond the scope of the argument to do so. Nor is it necessary to consider nice distinctions between psychology and the other social sciences. What does need consideration is how psychology sees its place in the world of knowledge, for implied in this will be how it sees its development and therefore to some extent its actual capacity for development. As the argument will be referred chiefly to the question of development, it will be sufficient to state an ordinary causal hypothesis of the systematic variety, which links the psychologist's perception of his task with the condition of psychology, and then to discuss the present consequences without taking much notice of historical causes.

In general, it could be said that, whether or not the psychologist is aware of it, he regards himself in much the same way as a natural scientist might have done a few decades ago. He regards himself as a dispassionate and disengaged observer of events which are external to him and which he can therefore observe or manipulate at will, in the same way as he can observe or manipulate events among things. And secondly, he regards himself as capable of elucidating the laws of behaviour of any field of activity, without reference, or without any but a reference on equal terms, to the laws of other branches of knowledge. Simply, he believes that psychology, which is a neutral branch of knowledge, contains in principle the laws of all human affairs: of history, art, letters, economics and sociology as well as of individual psychology.

Of course this is an over-simplification so gross that probably no psychologist has ever held these views exactly. On the other hand, both the assumption of neutrality and the reduction of all human affairs to individual psychology have been prominent enough in the development of psychology to have caused some distinctive features in that development. In order to show both that the over-simplification is not entirely false and that the views it misrepresents are incorrect, it will be sufficient to consider some of these distinctive developments.

PSYCHOLOGY IS NOT OUTSIDE SOCIETY

The reductive explanation of behaviour by referring it to facts of a lower level, or solely to a set of facts which is insufficient as a cause, has been noted already in various connections. Thus there is a slight tendency for some social psychologists to reduce behaviour to attitudes. The psychoanalysts' reduction of neurosis to the failure to achieve genital primacy (cf. Fenichel's account of analytic therapy [23, Ch. 23 and especially p. 572]) is well known, though, as Suttie [67, p. 216] argues, it is not evidently a sufficient explanation. Much greater reductions are involved in the empiricists' occasional direct equation of abstract with real behaviour and in the animal psychologist's similar occasional equation. On the larger scale which it is here relevant to consider, ingenious explanations in terms of individual psychology have been offered for substantial parts of history, art, sociology and theology. It is proposed to show, not that psychology has nothing to say about these, but that it has been trying to say the wrong things.

For this purpose it is convenient to take the case of theology, as explained by the psychoanalysts. In this, as in other examples to be discussed, there is of course no intention of giving a specially critical account of the work of the psychoanalysts. The example is taken merely because they are the pre-eminent pioneers of applications of psychological theory to a wide range of human affairs, so that their strength in extending psychology exposes them peculiarly to criticisms that simply do not apply to the less adventurous schools. Besides this, the example is particularly appropriate for, if there is any branch of knowledge which in the contemporary intellectual climate positively invites a reduction to individual psychology, and especially to psychopathology, it is theology.

The psychoanalysts' detailed reduction of theology derives from their general view that the Christian religion is a therapeutic cult. The side issues of this modern version of the Arian heresy and its counterpart, that psychology is an illegitimate religion, need not be considered. The first and most obvious consequence is that the psycho-analysts have somewhat odd views about what Christians believe. Thus Jones [33, p. 211] writes: 'As to the beliefs themselves, psycho-analytic investigation of the unconscious mental life reveals that they correspond closely with the phantasies of infantile life, mainly un-conscious ones, concerning the sexual life of one's parents and the conflicts this gives rise to.' Flugel [24, pp. 166–168, and Ch. 17] sets out similar views, as have various other psychoanalysts. The close correspondence which Jones alleges might have been less noticeable had he been better acquainted with Christian beliefs, so that it is possible that this and similar engaging speculations throw more light on why psychoanalysts do not believe than on why Christians do. In any case, if there were close correspondence the argument by analogy would show nothing by itself because, as Ricoeur observes [56, pp. 377–382], no activity can be regarded as only an elaboration of earlier and simpler activities. At all events, this reduction must be separately established and not merely assumed. With theology, this would require reference to history, for theology begins with a set of historical (that is, empirical and verifiable) propositions that have exactly the same status as any other historical propositions. This point is perhaps generally not known in learned circles, for Ayer [2, pp. 119–120], for example, writes off theological propositions as unverifiable when he apparently means only those of the more speculative parts of natural theology; dogmatic theology he has apparently not heard of. The psychoanalysts would thus be in good company if they did the same, but Jones, at least, is more aware of the historical basis of theology. The passage quoted above [33, p. 211] continues: 'The Christian story, an elaborate attempt to deal on a cosmic plane with these universal conflicts, can be fully accounted for on human grounds alone without the necessity of invoking super-natural intervention. Whether, nevertheless, such intervention took place as well must remain a matter of opinion, but the story itself is no proof of it.'

The difficulty is now apparent. The psychoanalyst finds himself incompetent to make a properly historical assessment of the his-torical propositions of theology, so he suspends judgement on these, while asserting that they are unnecessary to the explanation of theology. This presumably will depend on the argument by analogy, which will account for theology 'on human grounds alone' when it derives from the analyst's interpretation of Christian experience. It is a considerable weight for this analogical interpretation to carry, so that one might expect to find it more carefully made than it is, or even to find it done with the understanding due to personal experience. However, Christian belief is not possible experimentally. One can no more believe conditionally, with suspended judgement, than one can love conditionally or throw oneself completely into a task, or even undergo a successful psychoanalysis, conditionally. The psycho-analyst unfortunately has no recourse to experience that he can understand from within but, if he is still not altogether convinced by his analogical argument, he can sharpen it so as to rewrite history. This Jones does [33, p. 360] in his ingenious essay on the Holy Ghost:

'Not only must the Mother logically constitute the third member of any Trinity whose two other members are Father and Son, not only is this so in all the other numerous trinities known to us, but there is a considerable amount of direct evidence that this was originally so in the Christian myth itself.'

The detailed evidence that Jones refers to includes only three rather fragmentary sources, two of which are not Christian but gnostic and all of which are of uncertain date. Whether these should weigh against the numerous extended and apparently prior statements of the orthodox doctrine of the Holy Ghost is arguable: but it is not argued. It is the analogy, that Jones' view 'must logically' be correct that carries the weight of the argument. It is not unreasonable to call this procedure the rewriting of history, because the passage begs a whole library of historical questions about sources, dates, authorship and so on. This, finally, is the weakness of the analysts' reduction of theology. Its historical propositions are perfectly capable of de-tailed analysis, by persons with the appropriate professional training working to the standards of scholarship usual in any field of learning. An analogy is not a causal analysis, and no other analysis is relevant to the proof or disproof of these propositions, any more than it is relevant to the proof or disproof of historical propositions about the Seven Years War, the decline of the Spanish empire or the winner of last week's horse race. The reduction of historical propositions to propositions of any other order by analogy is a logical confidence trick which is meaningless, even if it is fashionable in some of its applications.

Similar reductions have been proposed by psychoanalytic writers in the fine arts, in sociology and in history. An example of the last may again be drawn, with due apologies for so taking advantage of his stimulating versatility, from Jones [32, pp. 684-685], who implies that the rise of mass production industry was in some sense assisted by the sublimation of anal erotism, which at the time was particularly repressed. Besides this kind of strictly historical reduction, some tendencies to a reduction of the complex to the simple are apparent in social psychology. Thus LaPiere and Farnsworth [37, p. 57] observe that types of behaviour which are called good or bad are defined entirely subjectively and locally, which is more than somewhat exaggerated even if the statement is rather artificially referred to the point of view of psychology alone. Ichheiser [29, Ch. 4] is concerned that marked disagreements between persons should not all be written off as prejudice without consideration of their content, and, while his concern may be exaggerated, there are traces of this writing off in the literature. Besides the examples discussed in Chapter 5, one might refer to the pioneer industrial work of Mayo and his associates, in which, as Miller and Form [46, pp. 78, 79] observe, what was described as alogical thinking was quite logical thinking in a different frame of reference.

The conclusion is that observations of individual behaviour, which may be highly pertinent as far as they go, cannot be simply added to explain group behaviour. The economic, social or political group is no more the simple sum of a number of individuals than history is the simple repetition of modes of individual behaviour, in which the present can be telescoped with the past. At all events, one can reasonably say that if the implicit presuppositions of simple addition and repetition are to be accepted they must be established by demonstration in the same way as the presupposition of addition from abstract to real behaviour. Meantime, psychology's place in the study of human affairs generally can be assumed to depend on its observance of the hierarchical order of these affairs.

The psychologist's assumption that he is a neutral and detached observer can now be considered. This is the logical counterpart of the reductive method of study for, if only individual psychology needs to be considered, the psychologist can study this without reference to considerations which are beyond his professional sphere. He can detach himself from the complexities of his world and let nothing but the data themselves guide his investigation or action.

Neutrality in this sense, however, is not possible even in the procedure for which it has most clearly been defined as necessary, the conduct of psychoanalysis. The analyst, Fenichel [23, p. 571] says, is a ' "mirror" that does nothing but show to the patient what he is doing'. This is true in so far as the analyst does not react emotionally to what the patient says, but he is bound to react selectively. He is not a passive reflector but, as Ricoeur [56, p. 376] puts it, 'une autre conscience dechiffreuse'.[1] His deciphering is an active interpretation guided both by psychoanalytic theory and by his personal system of values, which latter is open to at least partial determination by nontechnical considerations in so far as it must depend on his nonexpert understanding of the whole range of human affairs. Of course

[1] 'Another consciousness that decodes.'

205

he does not obtrude his personal values in making his interpretations, but they are bound to be perceived (or misperceived) by the patient as much in what he does not say and in when he says nothing, as in what he says. Baudouin [4, pp. 468–474] observes that the patient listens for what the analyst does not say and interprets it, and Caruso [8, p. 166] notes that this is inevitable once the patient is sensitized by transference.

There is no need to pursue the argument about whether or not the attempt to be neutral is therapeutically efficient. The point that matters is that even in psychoanalysis, in which neutrality should be easier to attain than in any other procedure except, perhaps, the more superficial procedures of client centred therapy, it is in fact unattainable. Further, it is unattainable not because analysis is directed to an end that concerns the patient, but simply because the analyst's perception of the situation is selective and his selection derives as much from his whole social involvement as it does from his strictly professional knowledge. Neutrality is therefore impossible in even the most detached and abstruse investigation. The psychologist can only propose hypotheses, adopt methods of investigation and draw conclusions that are within his frame of reference, which depends on his whole involvement with his society. In the very decision to investigate or not, his perception is selective. Thus the long predominance of a purely introspective psychology (which Mounier [47, p. 352] rather impolitely calls: 'cette psychologie de rentiers'[1]), the psychoanalysts' quasi-biological orientation, the dependence of industrial psychology on management's logic of efficiency and the social psychologists' tendency to confound customs with morality, are not examples of errors or bias, but only examples of the sociological setting and limitations of knowledge.

It follows that the simplest way of dealing with the social involvement of psychology is not to ignore it but to understand it, which is easy enough. Psychology is quite relevant to the study of human affairs on any scale provided that its hypotheses and conclusions take only their due rank in the order of knowledge. Thus the analogical hypothesis proposed in theology by Jones is irrelevant because it cannot explain history; but an alternative hypothesis about the actual historical records that he analogizes away would be quite in order. Further, although its investigation would require professional competence in history, palaeography and so on, it would be a psychological hypothesis (as all historical hypotheses are ultimately), only one of the right order. In the same way, it is quite in order for psychology to propose hypotheses about and to investigate economic and technological behaviour so long as its hypotheses are of the right

[1] 'This psychology of the well-off.'

order; that is, so long as they are about relations between persons through the explicitly described and organized media of machines, goods, money and so on.

There need be no difficulty, either, over the fact that the psychologist is not neutral in any stage of his work, from decision through action to conclusions. This means only that his engagement with his world is empirical, speculative and hypothetical, in the same way as for anyone else, and continuously so in all the fields of his activity. He is not a sort of schizophrenic compound of an expert at times and for some purposes and a citizen at other times; he is indivisibly both (and other things too) at all times, including in his professional work. This is most obviously true in the psychologist's decision to undertake or not to undertake a particular practical task for a public agency or a business organization, but it is equally true in less obvious cases. Even if the psychologist is in a position to investigate only problems that interest him, regardless of their immediate practical significance, his decision on which problem to investigate next and indeed his very decision to undertake such investigations at all, are necessarily made within his social frame of reference, whether or not that is the same as his society's. In all cases, he begins by making a general decision that such and such would be a good kind of thing to do; and this is a personal moral decision, of the same sort as everyone makes in the conduct of his affairs, and depending equally on general considerations (including empirically open possibilities) outside the scope of exact expert knowledge, even if these considerations are neither analysed nor even noticed. In framing hypotheses and in conducting an investigation the psychologist is less dependent on general considerations, but is never independent of them; and their influence on his formulation of conclusions may again be weighty. Of course his dependence on general considerations is no more a purely individual, unique, dependence than is his or anyone's dependence in daily life. A marked community of interest is to be expected in any professional body, as it is in any organized society, but there is no need to exaggerate this into an automatic (and therefore neutral) function. The psychologist has the same empirical freedom of engagement as everybody, so that the whole of his work, as well as the whole of his life, is in a sense a hypothesis.

PSYCHOLOGY IS NOT ONLY A SOCIAL TECHNIQUE

The argument can now be taken back to the question of the development of psychology. Clearly how it develops will depend quite a bit on how psychologists understand their social involvement. If psychology is a neutral and additive study, it will develop by the accumulation of somewhat unrelated (and perhaps unrelatable) particulars that are studied only in a limited frame of reference. The alternative would be that psychology should develop in systematic and coherent relation with other studies of human affairs. The point of the argument is to show how this might be done, for the possibility of psychology's being relevant to the conduct of affairs generally depends on its developing in the way stated. Here again, as in the choice between abstract and real laws in psychology, there may be an important choice to be made. It is not proposed to discuss on what grounds the choice should be made because it has just been argued that such questions are beyond the scope of psychology. It is necessary, however, to consider the nature of this hypothetical choice, for its connection with psychology's possible social functions might lead to mistaken ideas of what is in question.

There is no question, firstly, of correcting the errors made in the various reductive applications of psychology that were discussed above. Historically considered, these applications were not errors at all; they were hypotheses depending on observations of fact and applied within the frame of reference of their times. The observations need no correction and the applications need only removal to a more adequate frame of reference; that is, to a more general one, as that is now possible. It follows that there is certainly no question of replacing a frame of reference that belongs to the past with an equally limited alternative. To replace the management's logic of efficiency in industrial psychology by the workers' logic of collective protection, or to replace the 'bourgeois morality' of psychoanalysis by a theoretical system based on material acquisitiveness, would merely perpetuate the confusion of levels in the hierarchy of knowledge. It follows, again, that there is no question of discussing the present possible applications of psychology to social problems. Whatever the choice that might need considering is, it is not the choice between alternative brands of applied psychology.

Nor is there any question of suggesting clarification in the public position of psychology. It is true that the nature and functions of psychology are often popularly misunderstood, but there seem to be no serious consequences of this. The least misunderstanding is that caused by the occasional psychologist who makes public pronouncements, with apparent authority, in fields of which he is ignorant. Embarrassing as this may be, it is very rare compated to similar pronouncements by natural scientists, and can hardly be thought seriously to mislead the public. Then there is the public expectation that psychology is a kind of small-scale magic, which can solve all individual problems by changing the colour of the walls; and a similar belief may be developing, that psychology's large-scale magic will be able to solve all group, social and political problems by explaining them. Strictly as magical beliefs, these are the natural superstitions of a credulous age, in which it is prejudice to hold any firm beliefs except that firm belief is impossible. However, they do not seem likely to have any undesirable effect on the development of psychology. If they are elaborated and put into practice without regard to the limitations of psychology, they are likely to be rapidly discredited by failure; and if they are acted on, not as magic, but with an intelligent regard for the partiality and insufficiency of psychology, they can only assist its development.

Lastly, there is the occasional (but apparently growing) superstition that psychology offers unlimited possibilities for social control by manipulation, and this too seems to have no consequences of importance.

The choice, then, is not between a socially conscious and accepted psychology and one that is isolated from practical affairs and distrusted. It is simply between psychology developed in accordance with its own nature, as a coherent and wide-ranging body of knowledge which is integrated with the wider study of human affairs and a psychology which is a mere accumulation of particulars. On whatever grounds the choice between lines of development is made (and it may be as well to repeat that it would be irrelevant to discuss these), it is obviously relevant in the most general sense to the social functions of psychology, for its possible future functions will depend simply on how it is developed.

One could go further, and observe that the development of psychology as a broad empirical study is possible only in some societies. Psychology may have begun as an academic speculation but it quickly moved into the practical investigation of individual problems and maladjustment and thence into the investigation of group problems. It is a natural study in a society which is aware of its difficulties and can attend to them empirically for it is required by, and is only possible in, such a society. The retirement of German psychology after 1933 into academic isolation from practical affairs is an example of the impossibility of a seriously empirical psychology in a society which takes a fixed *a priori* view of its difficulties. In this connection, it may be noted that the rule of thumb applied psychology that was used in Germany for mass manipulation was also limited, for it had to be applied on top of extensive corruption and inefficiency in public administration and in industry. These fatal weaknesses were the price of the absolute state, which could no more expose them to the attention of psychology than it could afford simply to dispense with them. Judged by the total absence of social and industrial psychology in the ordinary sense (that is, field investigations) the condition of psychology in Russia is similar. Of course in the Marxist system social psychology is not a separate study but merely a branch of politics. However, descriptions of the heroic Soviet 'man (which appear in psychology texts as well as in popular sources: cf. Kornilov, Smirnov and Teplov [35]), do not seem altogether adequate as a causal analysis of the situation even when they are balanced by descriptions of the workers and so on who periodically fail in their duty or betray the country. Both the incidence and the origin of the latter need explanation; but, on the hypothesis adumbrated by Dicks [17], explanation is the last thing that could be done from within the system. It may be noted, finally, that the process described is not the only possible stultification of psychology. It would be quite possible to push the development of particular techniques of social manipulation (opinion polls used as propaganda, direct and indirect propaganda methods and so on) to the limit of their usefulness in a rigid society that depended only on the comparatively polite methods of group pressure and ostracism to ensure conformity to the pattern of the majority. However, this process would be little different in nature from the one first described. The limit of usefulness of short-run techniques would soon be reached, and the investigation of general problems (such as the long-run consequences of rigidity and conformity under group pressure) would be barred to psychology under pain of ostracism.

It may be concluded that the broad development of psychology is guaranteed in principle, not at all by its unlimited potential in social manipulation but by its intractability as a mere technique of manipulation. So far as it depends on the very nature of psychology, the main choice in development is not between immediately useful developments and remoter general ones, nor between developments for various kinds of application, nor between developments in different social interests. The choice is in the first place between a broad development, which alone would have a theoretical base sufficient for a wide range of applications and which is possible only in a society that is open to these applications, and a development by the mere accumulation of detail within the present framework of psychology, which would be capable of relatively few applications. If the broad development is undertaken, all the decisions about the detailed social involvement of psychology remain to be made, by reference to the wider field of human affairs. If development is only within the present framework, the more general questions hardly arise. The next step, then, is to ignore the almost infinite possibilities of proliferation in particular investigations in psychology, and to describe the general lines of development that might be sufficient to integrate it.

THE DEVELOPMENT OF PSYCHOLOGY

The first main line of development is to extend psychological investigation into new areas. As investigation has been concentrated on abstract behaviour, this means chiefly extending into the investigation of overt behaviour in real life situations of all kinds. This is already in progress, but is still a minor line of enquiry compared to the investigation of abstract behaviour. Further, it is important that overt behaviour should be carefully defined. What is necessary is to investigate not only what the person does as the experimenter sees him doing it, but especially what he does as he sees himself doing it. This opens an enormous field, as Krech and Crutchfield [36, p. 80] observe: 'Almost the entire task of obtaining a good description of the perceived social worlds of different people remains yet to be done.' It would therefore be necessary to pay special attention to behaviour from which covert intentional perceptions can be directly inferred and doubtless necessary to extend the enquiry where this inference was difficult or impossible. In principle, then, the enquiry would cover all behaviour in real life situations and, again in principle, it would be directed to the person's behaviour in all real life situations simultaneously. As a working convenience it might be necessary to study the behaviour of the worker, the parent, the voter and so on, but studies that begin by sectioning the person run the risk of lapsing into abstraction even if they are necessary for some special comparative enquiries.

An important extension within the study of real behaviour would be the special comparative study of a forgotten part of society, the working classes. Psychology, as a middle-class occupation, has depended so much on the study of middle-class persons that information about other persons is meagre. It is necessary information in all cases in which their perception of their social world might be different, for the mere assumption that it is not different is an example of the reduction of the complex to the simpler. Differences in general social ideology and in the perception of the home and family, of education and of work are obvious enough in common experience but largely remain to be explored by psychology.

Another important extension within the same main development would be the particular study of real behaviour in areas in which much work has already been done, child development and education. There are innumerable cross-sectional studies of changes with time in

211

children's abstract social behaviour, abilities and so on. Beyond the pioneer work of Isaacs and Piaget (which is too well known to require detailed reference) there are very few studies of the actual continuous development of social and intellectual behaviour in real life situations. The study of what the child does at home and at school, from the child's point of view, has been undertaken by Warner, Havinghurst and Loeb [71], Hollingshead [28], Oeser and Hammond [50] and Oeser and Emery [51], as well as others. But this work can only be said to have just begun if it is compared to the volumes of information available about children's scores on adjustment inventories and abstract tests of ability, achievement and so on.

Perhaps the likeliest case for studying a section of the person's life would be the study of sub-intentional and intellectual behaviour in real life situations, as these are not areas of behaviour but complex general modes which occur in all areas. Sub-intentional behaviour would include both articulate and fragmentary fantasies and both conscious and unconscious, or the floating and the submerged background of intentional behaviour, whether covert or overt. Real intellectual behaviour is the actual co-ordination and conceptual direction of overt behaviour. It certainly needs studying because very little is known about it after decades of intelligence testing; this work in the abstract field requires almost complete repetition in the field of real behaviour. However, whether it would be possible or economical to detach sub-intentional or intellectual behaviour from the intentional behaviour they respectively back up and co-ordinate, is not clear. It might be easier to study these kinds of behaviour in context, as they occur.

Lastly, it may be suggested that the study of history and of the exceptional (of all kinds) should be included in the extensions outlined, as a matter of course. The study of the person's history would be of special importance, for not very much is known about how the person learns under ordinary real life conditions, and especially about how he learns his major adjustments. The bald account given in Chapter 6 of the nature and conditions of learning is bald for this reason. The greater part of the investigations of learning has been directed to learning in artificial experimental situations or, at least, in situations much simpler than those of ordinary continued experience. Whether the extensive laws of learning derived from these specialized investigations would be capable of generalization, remains to be seen. It cannot be assumed that they would until the investigation of learning is extended.

Particular extensions of the field of psychology into the study of economics, sociology, history, the arts and so on (in order to clear up the confused findings in these fields that were discussed above) are not suggested because the general extension of the scope of psychology would include these automatically in due course.

These various extensions would enable psychology to avoid the reduction of complex processes, by analogy, to simpler ones by the direct study of the complex. They are not suggested, of course, as an immediately possible programme for psychology but only as hypothetically possible over a long period. The immediate possibilities of such extensions depend quite a bit on another kind of extension, into the comparative study of methods of enquiry. Even if hypotheses about these can be stated, not nearly enough is known about how they work in detail to ensure an economical choice of methods for general purposes. Much of the comparative study, however, could be done from data already in hand and beyond this it could easily be carried as a secondary investigation in any general enquiry. It would be necessary only to reflect the enquiry, as it were, so that it was directed to the comparison of findings by different methods as well as the comparison of findings about different persons.

The second main line of development in psychology would be the study of certain general questions which are now ignored or insufficiently noticed, and which, if they would require continuous investigation over a very long period, are none the less reasonably open to immediate attention.

The first of these questions is the relation of the experimenter to his subject, of the psychologist to the persons he studies or advises and so on. It may be that this is not a very special and distinctive personal relation, but to assume that it is essentially the same as any other practical or causal relation between persons might be to explain the complex by false analogy with the simple, for the psychologist deals largely with persons under stress who consult him because they are under stress. It certainly cannot be assumed that this relation is sufficiently explained by analogy with the scientist's handling of material. However right MacMurray [42, p. 111] may be in saying that psychology is purely instrumental, this is true only from the point of view of the psychologist who sees himself as a neutral observer or agent. What needs investigating is how the person sees the situation; what he expects of the psychologist, in what circumstances, how his perceptions change in the situation and so on.

This needs investigating even in the case of the almost neutral situation in which the psychologist seeks only information for general research purposes; for even here nothing can be done unless the person sees the situation as relevant to his purposes, and the conditions under which he will do so are not altogether obvious. Investigation of communication in situations in which the person has a considerable stake, ranging from simple vocational counselling through to the most extended psychotherapy, is much more necessary. Very little is known, anywhere in the range, of just how the parties' perceptions of each other and themselves develop as the series proceeds. In consequence, very little is known of the conditions under which different kinds of communication may be usefully initiated by the psychologist. In the simpler cases, at least (such as vocational counselling and counselling used merely for symptom reduction), the decision between offering a bare minimum of stimulating but non-committal comments, presenting a fair range of interpreted facts, and simply giving advice may be sufficiently supported by the psychologist's personal experience and skill but cannot be supported by reference to a systematic general treatment of the differences between these procedures because there is no such treatment.

The kind of investigation suggested would obviously be relevant to the question whether psychotherapy is of any use; in fact, it would enable this silly question to be tackled intelligently. That the question usually proposed is merely how many persons are discharged fit for duty after different kinds of treatment, is a natural consequence of the instrumental outlook of psychology, but it need not be accepted as final. As was argued in Chapter 7, the question of what persons learn in the course of treatment is more important. The investigation of the larger question would naturally require the consideration of all kinds of relations between the person and the experimenter, whether the latter was a psychotherapist, a psycho-surgeon, a general practitioner or anyone else. It would thus be similar to the investigation of a still larger question, that of the relation between the psychologist and the subject when the former is either a non-communicating authority or is, in a sense, the subject's agent. The difference between selection and counselling in education and in industry, for example, may depend only on practical convenience. On the other hand, it may have far reaching and important consequences in the differences in the results of these processes; and this could only be determined by enquiry.

The whole group of enquiries outlined would doubtless go on as long as psychology does and would be tedious in nature, as it would have to be conducted largely by inference from comparative studies of different relations. However, these practical difficulties are the more, rather than the less, reason for including such enquiries within the immediate scope of a broadly developing psychology.

A second and even more complex general question is that of the constitutional limits of learning, about which little is known in some important cases beyond the bare fact that there are limits. The most important case is that discussed in Chapter 7, the inherited predispositions (whatever they are) to learn abnormal behaviour.

Another possible case is the innate limits of intellectual learning. It is known that the learning required for solving intelligence test items is subject to innate limits but, as Eysenck [21, pp. 175, 176] observes, it does not necessarily follow that the limitation, which accounts for only a part of any one test performance, would be weighty for the sum of a number of tests. One could go a step further and observe that as the relation between real intellectual behaviour and intelligence test behaviour is unknown but apparently not close, the innate limits of learning real intellectual behaviour might be of either greater or less practical significance than those of learning abstract test behaviour. However, it is not clear that this question has as many implications for the general development of psychology as has the question of the inherited factor in mental disorder. Other possible investigations of the biological limits of learning seem to be clearly unimportant. Constitutional (not necessarily inherited) differences in glandular functions or in metabolism generally may or may not be related to general qualities of temperament such as energy, emotionality, restlessness and so on; but the investigation of this question could well be left until these general qualities have been defined by the psychological study of real behaviour. The case with the study of the person's instinctive behaviour, as suggested by Tinbergen [68, pp. 205–210], is different. The relation between the human instincts and learnt behaviour was studied for centuries before psychology was heard of and it does not seem that much could now be added to what is known. Tinbergen, indeed, suggests that behaviours such as scratching may be innate but this, however interesting it may be to a zoologist, is hardly a matter of importance for psychology.

The last and most complex general question that psychology might usefully keep in view, at least in its broad development, is the description and analysis of normal behaviour. To regard the normal as merely that which is statistically average, or generally accepted, or officially accepted, here and now but not necessarily there and then is to accept an unnecessary reduction of the scope of psychology. Psychology must describe the simple case before it can generalize to the complex but only a mistaken view of its neutrality confines it to the simple case. The study of what kinds of behaviour can vary from society to society or from time to time, and within what limits they can vary, is certainly within the scope of psychology. The elementary danger of transferring criteria of adjustment from one society to another need not be exaggerated. On this, Young [74, pp. 74, 75] reasonably observes that a pattern of maladjustment in one society may have a different function and significance in others. It follows that one cannot characterize societies by patterns drawn from one only. From Dicks' accounts [16, 17] of German and Russian modes of behaviour, for example, it would not be reasonable to infer (and Dicks does not) that German society was hypomanic and Russian society is schizophrenic. It could be inferred that some kinds of hypomanics or schizoids would be better adjusted in some positions in these societies than they would in other societies. But it could be inferred equally that incoherent manics and catatonic schizophrenics would be as badly adjusted there as anywhere. The impossibility of simple transfer between societies does not mean that no generalization is possible. On the contrary, the study of particular variations and their conditions would be expected to lead to the inference of general laws of variation, including not only what does vary from place to place or time to time but also what does not. The latter in turn would include both the kinds of behaviour which are maladjusted in any known or even in any imaginable society and the kinds of accepted behaviour which are necessary for the continuance of any known or imaginable society. The limits of the impossible, the acceptably variable and the minimum invariable are all open to empirical study and description within the framework of human affairs generally (including history).

It would seem, indeed, that there may be enough evidence already to support some generalizations about normality that would go a little further than the mere parallel description of different modes of normal adjustment. Young's summary [74, pp. 50–55] of the general modes of adjustment of eight primitive societies shows that there are considerable differences among these societies, and concomitant differences in the nature and degree of the maladjustments commonly found in them. A comparison among these societies or of these with civilized societies, on the basis of the survival value under natural or social stress of their modes of adjustment, might well be too hypothetical to be worth attempting. But a comparison on the basis of their common maladjustments would be easy, for these evidently differ both in their nature and in their degree or incidence. Tension within the person, that is to say, differs in its derivation and strength from one society to another; so that it should be possible to establish (for example) whether cannibals or head-hunters are more or less torn by incompatible inner strivings than socially mobile persons or unwilling spinsters. These might or might not be possible comparisons, for generalizations about large historical conjuctions are open to doubt; and, if they were possible, they might or might not be important to psychology. Neither question can be answered until they are attempted. Psychology, that is to say, might well study human nature in general as well as in particular. Of course it is not suggested that this would be a substitute for the study of morality.

Fromm's attempt [25] to construct a naturalistic system of ethics fails, not so much because of the inevitable insufficiency of his evidence about human nature in general, as because he has no ground for making the implied transfer from description to prescription. The person's empirical freedom of engagement in prescribing for himself (or in accepting a prescription) does not oblige him to take into account considerations beyond psychology but it certainly allows him to do so. The broadest and most general description of human nature as it is and was could not, therefore, be a sufficient guide to action by itself but it would be considerably more relevant than is a description of abstract particulars only.

This last point suggests a conclusion. The coherent development of psychology, as outlined above, into a general body of knowledge to which the name psychology clearly belongs is one possibility. The most sharply contrasted possibility would be the development of psychology by the accumulation of detail. In this, behaviour in real life situations would be studied only in so far as the developing speciality of social psychology managed to maintain its position; and then only in so far as it managed to avoid falling into abstraction. The methods of psychology would develop only in further refinements of the experimental procedures which put psychology through the motions of a natural science. Lastly, the general problems of psychology would remain unnoticed, for it would be quite logical for the description of normality as a set of averages on abstract measures to include the prescription in applied psychology (in psychotherapy as well as in all other fields of application) of an endless catalogue of indiscriminately derived nostrums. It is not suggested that this kind of development would be inferior to the coherent development described, or that the latter should be preferred, accepted and undertaken. The decision, in principle, between the two kinds of development is very clearly one of the decisions that must be made with reference to many much wider considerations than just the difference between the two kinds. The description of this difference does not determine the decision, it merely enables a decision on more clearly known grounds.

CONCLUSION

THE whole discussion of the nature of psychology may be summed up by returning to the practical difficulties and differences of approach that were set out in the Introduction. Part of the difficulty of handling even a fairly simple case in the practice of applied psychology may be that it has to be understood, ultimately, as a singular case; and the development of the laws of psychology can never altogether remove this difficulty. However, it is to some extent true that present difficulties are due merely to psychology's immaturity. But some difficulties are clearly due to the nature of psychology, which at the present seems to be developing so as to cut itself off deliberately from life. In this development, common experience is left outside the laboratory or test room and the psychologist studies only what can be simply defined, manipulated as an object, and measured, so that he can deduce laws which are exact even if they are irrelevant to human behaviour.

This development may be only the latest consequence of the analytic approach which has long been usual in psychology, but it is not altogether clear why this approach remains popular. The addition axiom on which it depends assumes, at the least, that the functional relations of processes can be inferred from the study of the isolated processes. It is not necessary to make the doubtfully meaningful assertion that the whole is greater than the sum of its parts to discredit this assumption. Experience of the simplest machine or organism or sequence of behaviour is sufficient to show that the study of isolated components or processes can go no further than the inference of possible functional relations which may or may not be actual. Of course the study of isolated processes, or fragmentary behaviour, may be necessary; but the analytic approach, in falsely proposing it as the sole necessity, does something which is not even economical, for fragments of behaviour could just as well be studied in their context, as they occur. The analytic approach is most doubt-

218

CONCLUSION

ful when it goes to the extreme of asserting that the fragments to be added are fragments of behaviour in purely artificial situations. In this case the addition axiom includes the radical assumption that the functional relations of the real processes which are not studied can be inferred from the study of certain isolated processes which are not known to resemble real processes and in some cases are obviously quite dissimilar. This is rather like a zoologist's assuming that he can infer a monkey's functional economy from the histological study of various fish tissues; and the time may well come when the study of the electronic computer is made to stand for the study of the man who invented it. In its extreme form, the addition axiom is so fantastic that one can no longer regard it as merely the support of an analytic approach which has been naturally, if perhaps unfortunately, prominent in psychology. The position is no longer that psychology proposes to build up from the bottom, limited as that procedure has been, but that psychology proposes to build its own private world.

It seems, indeed, that psychology is tending to be involved in the positivistic retreat from life. What is meaningful, what can be studied, is what anybody without any special competence can understand after a few minutes' reflection, or a few days' study, or a few weeks' experimenting. The logically tidy and the easily abstractable are not to be taken as the real universe, for there are as many real universes as there are different points of view among observers; but the simple and easily understood are to be given an absolute priority as objects of study. Complex events, that can be defined and studied only by prolonged work, are to be set aside because, at the best, they are too hard for science to investigate and, at the worst, they are not open to scientific investigation; they are the mere emotional froth on, or the disorderly surface of, the tidy little world of simple abstractions. If this drastic simplification of life is accepted, the way is open for psychology to abandon any pretence of relating its findings to real life. Job adequacy, marital adjustment, neuroticism and so on are what various tests measure. They are operationally defined. That they have little or nothing to do with the person's ordinary behaviour outside the test room is immaterial. The approach is no longer analytic, it is simply and purely abstract. One present reaction to the relative lack of success of the analytic approach (except in certain special fields) may be to turn to the direct study of ordinary behaviour. The other, and perhaps the more marked, reaction is to turn away from reality and to set about constructing a whole psychology of the artificial.

To call this a schizophrenic reaction would be a statement of the wrong order, for the phenomenon is social rather than individual.

219

One way of coping with the complex unpleasantness of a disordered society is to ignore it and to retreat into a private world of endless ritual play. What the harassed citizen does with his meaningless work and his frantic leisure the positivist does in a more sophisticated way with his endless analyses of invented behaviour. But it is merely his misfortune that he thinks what he is doing is psychology. The only ground for confining psychology to the study of quizzes, muscle tremors and puzzle boxes is that some persons do not like studying anything but these; which is no ground at all. It is on this account that certain topics which are conventionally important in psychology have been little discussed. In the conventional sense, experimental psychology means the study of the person's reaction to mechanical instruments, and the psychology of learning means the study of the person learning nonsense syllables or learning the layout of a maze. It is unfortunately true that little empirical investigation has been done outside the field of simple controllable events; but the conventional view that this field is fundamental for psychology depends only on a personal preference for studying the abstract.

This account doubtless exaggerates both the prominence and the weaknesses of the abstract movement in psychology, in order to make the point that this movement is a reflection of a common social phenomenon. This point is supported by the consideration of the other quasi-schizophrenic reaction to the complexities of a disordered society; the declaration, in the more sophisticated sections of literature and the arts, that existence is at the least purely private and at the worst unintelligible, absurd or terrifying. Even the more extreme forms of this declaration would be of use to psychology in so far as they pointed to the complexity of common experience. In any form, of course, the declaration goes too far. To say that common experience is complex and is ultimately singular (the direct knowledge of the existent) is useful, but to say that experience is chaotic because it cannot be generalized by abstraction at all is, again, only to declare a personal preference which can in no way define the nature of psychology. However, if this preference would simply make empirical psychology impossible, it is complementary to the positivist's preference. The individualistic artist agrees with the positivist in finding that life, as he looks at it, is chaotic and meaningless; but the one goes on to exult in the anarchy of existence while the other withdraws discreetly into a private world of order.

Now it seems that most persons do not find it necessary to limit their knowledge either to that of bare existence or to that of the bare abstract concept. In common experience, there seems to be no difficulty in knowing the singular concrete being as an example, but

220

not only an example, of the general; or, to put it the other way round, in knowing the general as including, but not completely including, the diversity of the concrete. It would therefore seem natural for psychology to avoid the two anarchies of purely abstract order and pure disorder by accepting its derivation from common experience. In its nature, psychology is not a science but a history; or, if there is some magic in the word science, then psychology can be called a science in the general sense or a historical science, but not a natural science. It does not study events which are accessible only to special instruments and under special conditions. It studies what everyone knows, inevitably and as a matter of course, only it studies this with special care. Collingwood [13, p. 7] exaggerates the ease of knowing oneself in saying that everyone can know himself completely by reflection. Elsewhere he shows that this is not to be taken, however, as a simple process. He remarks [14, p. 219] that all knowledge of oneself is historical knowledge which is obtained by reflective re-enactment; and this is much the same as his description [14, pp. 249–281] of how ordinary historical evidence is gathered by inference, not observation. If this means only that psychology is a history, it could equally be taken to mean that history is psychology in its most general form. Whichever way the proposition is put, it would follow that, if history is difficult because of the remoteness of the events to be re-enacted, then psychology is likely to be at least as difficult because of the excessive variety of the events to be re-enacted; and perhaps, indeed, *because* of their nearness, if it is a matter of understanding oneself.

But there is no need to exaggerate or to misunderstand the specialization of psychology by assimilating it to the natural sciences. In the sciences, difficulties in formulating exact hypotheses, in testing them and in communicating findings are due to the extreme specialization of experience on which any science depends. It follows that the sciences, if they are universally valid, cannot be universally known. The scientific propositions which Stevens [66, p. 27] says are agreed upon by members of society are understood, and in that sense agreed upon, only by the members of small and highly specialized groups: everyone else accepts them on trust because he cannot possibly understand them, let alone test them.

In psychology, the difficulties of community in knowledge (from formulating hypotheses through to communicating findings) derive only from the fact that life is too short for anyone to study experience comprehensively. Anyone may have had, or could have, or at the least could imagine, the experience that psychology studies. Of course, in practice the study of common experience may be little more open to everyone than is the study of the special experience of the sciences.

In both cases, study requires intelligence, training, steady application and some degree of adventurousness. But psychology does not have to go and get experience and to use apparatus to take it apart. The experience is there, and is studied by reflection. As in the sciences, this may be a special kind of reflection, carried out only by special persons. But the object is universal and given, as it is not in the sciences; and if psychology is to deserve its name it cannot abandon this object for the irrelevant pursuit of the special and artificial. A psychology that does study its natural object is simply a specialization of common experience, or a specially intense concentration of study within common experience. The psychologist is then not a detached observer of events over which he has full control. He is a person who is empirically free to discover the common determination of experience in a common engagement with other persons who are equally free. Similarly, the psychologist does not fix his attention only on those hypotheses that can be tidily circumscribed in space or time. He accepts it as a consequence of his empirical freedom of engagement that these hypotheses, necessary as they may be, are merely components of larger hypotheses which may be testable only in the whole of his life, or, indeed, in the whole of history in so far as history is itself a hypothesis.

This follows from the simple fact that, as Farrer [22, p. 243] says, we know ourselves directly and know all other beings only by analogy, in increasing remoteness as we pass from knowing other persons to knowing inanimate objects. That is why the use of biological, mechanical, physical and diagrammatic models in psychology is doubtful. The most that we know of the general properties of things may be best expressed as if these were the general properties of constructs or models. But the general properties of persons are known from within, and are best stated by analogy with persons; that is, with themselves. There are degrees of knowledge and it is not merely unnecessary but wrong to reduce all knowledge to the lowest degree. The proper basis for a realistic psychology is common experience. This is the proper source of general information and hypotheses which can be tested by special investigation and developed into laws; and these are properly formulated and tested by reference back to common experience. For the most part common experience appears in psychology only when the psychologist lapses rather unhappily into anecdotes for lack of scientific evidence or into practical judgment for lack of a rigorous measurement technique. In this respect, Allport's [1] open and sustained reference to common experience is exceptional. But, however unfashionable it may be, this reference is necessary. It does not destroy, but guarantees, the special status of psychology; for although psychology is

222

not simply common experience written out in special words, it is and can only be common experience extended, clarified and corrected by special procedures.

It is evident that psychology has already been successful in extension, clarification and correction, not only in the simple extension of information which there is no time to gather in ordinary circumstances, but especially in cases where it has been able to show that the person is not quite such a simple object as might be commonly supposed. Psychology demonstrated long since that even seeing, remembering and thinking are by no means as simple and straightforward as common experience may take them to be; and followed this up by showing that these processes are selective in accordance with the person's social purposes. As far as it has gone, the study of development and of social behaviour has shown equally that the person is not quite as simple as might be imagined. Applied psychology, in the study of techniques of child rearing, classroom techniques and industrial management methods, has shown that the person is not merely a receptacle to be filled with food, knowledge or morale. There is no need to give more examples. Many more could be given, but it must be allowed that, altogether, they would establish the promise of psychology more firmly than its performance. Psychology has gone little beyond common experience in establishing the general ordinary causal laws of behaviour, while it has established some component and many abstract laws. This is not remarkable, for psychology in what might be called its classical phase has been more concerned with establishing its position and finding a basis of work than with broad investigation. The only account one can give for ordinary causal laws is largely speculative and hypothetical; and the whole point of this account is to show how psychology could develop these into firmly established laws by building on common experience instead of moving progressively away from it.

In this development psychology would of course change its relations with philosophy by abandoning its reliance on the fashionable epistemology of the sciences. It is true, as Collingwood [12, pp. 105, 106] says, that philosophical judgement means knowing something better which one knows already. It is also true that what the philosopher knows includes what is reported by any special investigator, the scientist among others. But in principle this includes everything in human behaviour and not only the simple, almost fragmentary, intellectual operations that are the sole interest of many philosophers. An abstract artificial psychology is the natural counterpart of a philosophy thus reduced. Both equally ignore those major properties of life which Ichheiser [29, Ch. 1] says are too large and obvious to be noticed, not only because they are large and obvious but probably also because attending to them would require an undesired involvement with the complexity of ordinary life.

If the psychologist prefers his present philosophical partnership to the limitations of an introspective philosophical psychology, he merely exchanges a bad hindrance to his activities for a worse. What one might call philosophical anthropology begins where empirical psychology ends; or, conversely, empirical psychology studies the particular within the universal field of philosophical anthropology, and thus returns to philosophy a realistic account of the diversity of persons. But this partnership is possible only if neither philosophy nor psychology is restricted to the barely human field of experience of the quasi-physical. That psychology, at least, need not be thus restricted is given in the fact that it is at the end of its classical phase. Its development from the analysis of special functions towards the study of pure abstractions has been by no means as simple as the exaggerated account given above suggests; but it is, on the whole, true that psychology has reached a critical point at which it must enter the next phase of its development. In this phase, the chief and sharply divergent possibilities are either a development into increasing abstraction from life or an open development on the basis of common experience.

It need hardly be said that this conclusion is meant to be only a description of the situation and not a criticism. The argument that the situation is ripe for a possible change of direction may well appear critical, merely by the omission of a detailed appreciation of psychology's earlier direction. But it would be a historical absurdity to criticize psychology for having developed so far in accordance with its nature and its situation in the world of learning; and no such absurdity is intended. The description of the present situation is meant only to show that this now makes possible certain different lines of development. The description of these lines is a hypothesis about the whole body of professional experience which psychologists might have under certain conditions. It is thus no more a prescription for action, let alone a prediction, than it is a criticism; for, as a hypothesis, it refers to circumstances that may or may not be capable of realization in practice, and that cannot be specified so exactly as to determine action even in hypothetical circumstances. Besides that it would be presumptuous for anyone to prescribe the future of psychology, it is impossible to do this from within psychology. Even if the general argument is correct, the issue remains open, for the decision between abstract and realistic psychology must be made on wider grounds than are given merely in psychology itself.

A simpler consideration is that any development in psychology must be limited by the exigencies of the present situation. In any case, development can only be based on what has been done already. An argument which looks to the future can hardly do even the most elementary justice to the past; but one must be clear that the development of psychology has not only laid a general foundation for the next stage, whatever that may be, it has also gone far into detailed practical applications. The greater part of psychological work is in the established fields of application in clinical, educational and industrial psychology. These will obviously absorb more and more workers, but these workers will hardly be able to undertake major developmental projects. Research in psychology does not require special premises or costly equipment, so that it not only can but should be undertaken mainly by the working psychologist. Unfortunately, it does require time and staff, and one can hardly hope that the employers of working psychologists will see the point that basic research is an essential occupation for their employees. The main work of development must therefore be done elsewhere, by the few psychologists who are fortunate enough to be able to take it on. But they are, in fact, far fewer than would be adequate even for development on established lines. The established fields of application still require plenty of detailed developmental work, even if no new lines in these fields are explored. Besides this, psychology's firm identification as an emergency procedure guarantees support for the particular investigation of problems (and some pseudo-problems) rather than for general developmental work. It may not be easy to finance research into the problems of delinquency, old age, comics, backward children, gifted children, morale, fatigue, equipment design and so on, but it is much easier to do this than to finance research which is aimed simply at elucidating the ordinary causal laws of behaviour. This is somewhat paradoxical, for in psychology it is the basic research which would be directly and immediately relevant to practical problems. Basic research is not, as it is in the sciences, far removed from common experience; it is the specialized investigations that tend to be abstract and remote. However, if the analogy with the relation between science and technology reverses the situation in psychology, it is none the less likely to go on being applied.

Finally, the exigencies of the present situation must be met even in the teaching of psychology. It might be desirable to emphasize psychology's derivation from, or specialization within, common experience, and therefore to emphasize the scientific methods of enquiry which are proper to psychology rather than those of the natural sciences. But these would be changes of occasional emphasis only, as the main weight of teaching must obviously be carried by the systematic work that has been done, and most of this is specialized, if not abstract. It is not even possible, for example, to remove social psychology from its logically absurd place as a special subject and to put it in the centre of the psychology course because it is still only a specialization. The one change that might be possible in the present situation is to extend the practical teaching of skills in the personal relation of experimenter and subject. It is not suggested that the psychology course should include detailed training in a variety of diagnostic, survey, test and counselling techniques. The details are appropriately learnt in practice, on the job. But psychology, of all subjects, cannot be taught merely out of books, whether these are experimenters' manuals or general texts. The psychologist is, first and last, someone who sits down with somebody else and engages with him in a specialized kind of common task. The least the teacher can do is to show the student how this is done in general and to help him practice doing it.

REFERENCES

1. ALLPORT, GORDON W. *Personality. A Psychological Interpretation.* New York. Henry Holt and Co. 1937.
2. AYER, ALFRED JULES. *Language, Truth and Logic.* London. Victor Gollancz Ltd. 1951.
3. BAKKE, E. W. *The Unemployed Man.* London. Nisbet and Co. Ltd. 1933.
4. BAUDOUIN, CH. In symposium, Médecine, quatrième pouvoir? ed. by Em. Mounier. *Ésprit.* 1950, 165, 337–537.
5. BENEDICT, RUTH. *Patterns of Culture.* London. George Routledge and Sons. 1935.
6. BRITTON, KARL. *Communication.* London. Kegan Paul. 1939.
7. CAMERON, NORMAN. *The Psychology of Behaviour Disorders.* Boston. Houghton Mifflin. 1947.
8. CARUSO, IGOR A. *Psychoanalyse und Synthese der Existenz.* Vienna. Verlag Herder. 1952.
9. CATTELL, RAYMOND B. *Personality.* New York. McGraw-Hill. 1950.
10. CÉSARI, PAUL. *Les Déterminismes et les Êtres.* Paris. J. Vrin. 1938.
11. CHEIN, ISIDOR. 'The genetic factors in a-historical psychology.' *J. Gener. Psychol.* 1947, 36, 151–172.
12. COLLINGWOOD, R. G. *An Essay on Philosophical Method.* Oxford. Clarendon Press. 1933.
13. COLLINGWOOD, R. G. *The New Leviathan.* Oxford. Clarendon Press. 1942.
14. COLLINGWOOD, R. G. *The Idea of History.* Oxford. Clarendon Press. 1951.
15. CRONBACH, LEE J. *Essentials of Psychological Testing.* New York. Harper. 1949.
16. DICKS, HENRY V. 'Personality traits and National Socialist ideology.' *Hum. Rel.* 1950, 3, 111–154.
17. DICKS, HENRY V. 'Observations on contemporary Russian behaviour.' *Hum. Rel.* 1952, 5, 111–175.
18. DUFRENNE, M., and RICOEUR, P. *Karl Jaspers et la Philosophie de l'Existence.* Paris. Éditions du Seuil. 1947.
19. ECCLES, J. C. *The Neurophysiological Basis of Mind.* Oxford. Clarendon Press. 1953.
20. EYSENCK, H. J. *The Dimensions of Personality.* London. Routledge and Kegan Paul. 1947.

21. EYSENCK, H. J. *The Scientific Study of Personality.* London. Routledge and Kegan Paul. 1952.
22. FARRER, AUSTIN. *Finite and Infinite.* London. Dacre Press. 1943.
23. FENICHEL, OTTO. *The Psychoanalytic Theory of Neurosis.* London. Kegan Paul. 1946.
24. FLUGEL, J. C. *Man, Morals and Society.* London. Duckworth. 1945.
25. FROMM, ERICH. *Man for Himself.* London. Routledge and Kegan Paul. 1949.
26. GILSON, ÉTIENNE. *L'Être et l'Essence.* Paris. J. Vrin. 1948.
27. HEBB, D. O. *The Organisation of Behaviour. A Neurophysiological Theory.* New York. Wiley. 1949.
28. HOLLINGSHEAD, A. B. *Elmtown's Youth.* New York. Wiley. 1949.
29. ICHHEISER, GUSTAV. 'Misunderstandings in human relations.' *Amer. J. Sociol. Monog. Sup.* 1949, 55, 1–70.
30. JAQUES, ELLIOTT. *The Changing Culture of a Factory.* London. Tavistock Publications Ltd. 1951.
31. JASPERS, KARL. *Philosophie.* Band II, *Existenzerhellung.* Berlin. Julius Springer. 1932.
32. JONES, ERNEST. *Papers on Psycho-Analysis.* London. Baillière, Tindal and Cox. 1920.
33. JONES, ERNEST. *Essays in Applied Psycho-Analysis.* London. The Hogarth Press Ltd. 1951.
34. KALLMANN, FRANZ J. 'The Genetic Theory of Schizophrenia.' In Kluckhohn, Clyde, and Murray, Henry A. (Eds.) *Personality in Nature, Society and Culture.* New York. Alfred A. Knopf. 1949.
35. KORNILOV, K. N., SMIRNOV, A. A., and TEPLOV, B. M. *Psychology.* London. Society for Cultural Relations with the U.S.S.R. 1950.
36. KRECH, DAVID R., and CRUTCHFIELD, RICHARD S. *Theory and Problems of Social Psychology.* New York. McGraw-Hill. 1948.
37. LAPIERE, RICHARD T., and FARNSWORTH, PAUL R. *Social Psychology.* New York. McGraw-Hill. 1942.
38. LEWIN, KURT. *Principles of Topological Psychology.* New York. McGraw-Hill. 1936.
39. LEWIN, KURT. 'The Nature of Field Theory.' In Marx, Melvin H. (Ed.) *Psychological Theory: Contemporary Readings.* New York. MacMillan. 1951.
40. MCCLELLAND, DAVID C. *Personality.* New York. William Sloane Associates. 1951.
41. MACIVER, R. M. *Social Causation.* Boston. Ginn and Co. 1942.
42. MACMURRAY, JOHN. *The Boundaries of Science. A Study in the Philosophy of Psychology.* London. Faber and Faber. 1939.
43. MAIER, NORMAN R. F. *Principles of Human Relations.* New York. Wiley. 1952.
44. MARX, MELVIN H. 'The General Nature of Theory Construction.' In Marx, Melvin H. (Ed.) *Psychological Theory: Contemporary Readings.* New York. MacMillan. 1951.
45. MEAD, GEORGE H. *Mind, Self and Society.* Chicago University Press. 1946.

46. MILLER, D. C., and FORM, W. H. *Industrial Psychology*. New York. Harper. 1951.
47. MOUNIER, EMMANUEL. *Traité du Caractère*. Paris. Éditions du Seuil. 1947.
48. MURRAY, HENRY A. *Explorations in Personality*. New York. Oxford University Press. 1938.
49. NANSEN, ODD. *Day after Day*. London. Putnam and Co. Ltd. 1949.
50. OESER, O. A., and HAMMOND, S. B. (Eds.) *Social Structure and Personality in a City*. London. Routledge and Kegan Paul. 1954.
51. OESER, O. A., and EMERY, F. E. *Social Structure and Personality in a Rural Community*. London. Routledge and Kegan Paul. 1954.
52. OESER, O. A. (Ed.) *Teacher, Pupil and Task*. London. Tavistock Publications Ltd. 1955.
53. OGDEN, C. K., and RICHARDS, I. A. *The Meaning of Meaning*. London. Kegan Paul. 1946.
54. PARSONS, TALCOTT, and SHILS, EDWARD A. (Eds.) *Toward a General Theory of Action*. Cambridge, Mass. Harvard University Press. 1952.
55. PILGRIM TRUST. *Men Without Work. A Report to the Pilgrim Trust*. Cambridge University Press. 1938.
56. RICOEUR, PAUL. *Philosophie de la Volonté*. Tome 1, *Le Volontaire et l'Involontaire*. Paris. Aubier, Éditions Montaigne. 1949.
57. ROETHLISBERGER, F. J., and DICKSON, WILLIAM J. *Management and the Worker*. Cambridge, Mass. Harvard University Press. 1947.
58. RYLE, GILBERT. *The Concept of Mind*. London. Hutchinson's University Library. 1949.
59. SCHELER, MAX. *Wesen und Formen der Sympathie*. Bonn. Verlag von Friedrich Cohn. 1926.
60. SHELDON, RICHARD C. 'Some observations on theory in social science.' In Parsons, Talcott, and Shils, Edward A. (Eds.) *Toward a General Theory of Action*. Cambridge, Mass. Harvard University Press. 1952.
61. SHERIF, MUZAFER. *An Outline of Social Psychology*. New York. Harper. 1948.
62. SKINNER, B. F. *The Behaviour of Organisms*. New York. Appleton-Century Co. Inc. 1938.
63. SNYGG, DONALD, and COMBS, ARTHUR W. *Individual Behaviour*. New York. Harper. 1949.
64. SPENCE, KENNETH W. 'Types of constructs in psychology.' In Marx, Melvin H. (Ed.) *Psychological Theory: Contemporary Readings*. New York. MacMillan. 1951.
65. STEPHENSON, WILLIAM. *The Study of Behaviour: Q-Technique and its Methodology*. Chicago University Press. 1953.
66. STEVENS, S. S. 'Psychology and the science of science.' In Marx, Melvin H. (Ed.) *Psychological Theory: Contemporary Readings*. New York. MacMillan. 1951.
67. SUTTIE, IAN D. *The Origins of Love and Hate*. London. Kegan Paul. 1935.
68. TINBERGEN, N. *The Study of Instinct*. Oxford University Press. 1951.
69. TOLMAN, EDWARD C. 'The intervening variable.' In Marx, Melvin H.

(Ed.) *Psychological Theory: Contemporary Readings.* New York. MacMillan. 1951.

70. VITELES, MORRIS S. *Industrial Psychology.* New York. W. W. Norton and Co. Inc. 1932.

71. WARNER, W. L., HAVINGHURST, R. J., and LOEB, M. B. *Who shall be Educated?* London. Kegan Paul. 1946.

72. WISDOM, J. O. *Foundations of Inference in Natural Science.* London. Methuen and Co. Ltd. 1952.

73. WOODWORTH, ROBERT S., and SCHLOSBERG, HAROLD. *Experimental Psychology.* London. Methuen and Co. Ltd. Third edition. 1954.

74. YOUNG, KIMBALL. *Handbook of Social Psychology.* London. Kegan Paul. 1946.

INDEX

231

Russia, psychology in, 210, 216
Ryle, G., 16, 22, 26, 200

Scheler, M., 62
schizophrenia, schizoid character, 7, 40, 41, 75, 76, 93, 95, 122, 123, 156, 157, 176, 179, 180, 183, 216
Schlosberg, H., 107, 132
science, laws in, 170, 173, 199, 221
sentence-completion tests, 120
Sheldon, R. C., 144
Sherif, M., 50, 53, 54, 60, 63, 65, 86, 118, 160, 162, 196
Shils, E. A., 49, 60, 63, 69, 74
single event, the, 160
singularity, of the person, 159-62, 172, 197, 198, 200, 218, 220
Skinner, B. F., 31, 32
Smirnov, A. A., 210
Snygg, D., 15, 58, 92, 101
social psychology, 1, 5-8, 54, 65, 78, 79, 92, 108, 176, 200, 202, 206, 217, 226
Spence, K. W., 93, 186
staged situation, as method, 92, 114-116, 140, 141
statistical abstraction, 147-52
Stephenson, W., 196
Stevens, S. S., 22, 37, 44, 170, 221
stress, behaviour under, 160-2, 213
sub-intentional behaviour, 121, 122, 124, 126, 132, 134, 158, 181, 212
substantial abstraction, 102, 103, 106, 108, 120, 121, 124, 126, 131, 132, 134, 145, 146, 187
Suttie, I. D., 61, 202

synthetic abstraction, 102, 103, 106, 108, 110
synthetic judgements, 167, 168

tension, 56-9, 65, 216
Teplov, B. M., 210
Thematic Apperception Test, 120, 122, 142, 143, 168
theology, 171, 202, 203, 206
things, engagement with, 191, 192
Tinbergen, N., 26, 30, 160, 215
Tolman, E. C., 186
topology, 193
transferability, of findings, 25, 31-5, 39, 98, 102, 110, 111, 113, 115, 116, 119-21, 124, 127-9, 131, 138, 143, 146, 179, 188, 195

unconscious, the, 27, 29, 30, 94, 97, 121, 181
usefulness of laws in psychology, 174-6, 178, 179, 183, 187, 188, 194

validity, of tests, 163
verification, 10, 36-40, 43, 46
Viteles, M. S., 130
vocational counselling, guidance, selection, 2-4, 40, 92, 96, 113, 213, 214

Warner, W. L., 212
Wisdom, J. O., 170
Woodworth, R. S., 107, 132
word-association tests, 120, 144, 168
working classes, study of, 211

Young, K., 215, 216